# The ⑦ Energies of the Soul

# The ⑦ Energies of the Soul

Awaken Your Inner
**Creator, Healer, Warrior, Lover,
Artist, Explorer, & Master**

## DAVID GANDELMAN

Hier◉phantpublishing

Cover design by Laura Beers
Cover art by ©Creations/Shutterstock
Print book interior design by Frame25 Productions

Hierophant Publishing
San Antonio, TX
www.hierophantpublishing.com

If you are unable to order this book from your local
bookseller, you may order directly from the publisher.

Library of Congress Control Number: 2021949056

ISBN: 978-1-950253-19-7

10 9 8 7 6 5 4 3 2 1

# Contents

# Introduction

## First Steps

At sixteen, I was leading an American suburban teenage life—playing ice hockey, trying to date, and screwing around with my friends—until the day my brother came home from college and dragged me to a bookstore. He had been experimenting with, let's say, "mind-altering substances," and he wanted me to open my mind. He also thought that I was lazy and never read anything. So he forced me to choose a book.

Randomly—but, looking back, synchronistically—I picked up a book by spiritual teacher Eckhart Tolle called *The Power of Now* (New World Library, 1999). After reading just a few pages about how our minds are constantly lost to the past and the future, causing us miss the present moment, something deep in my consciousness shifted. It was as if I had been asleep in a dark room my entire life, hypnotized by the pull of time, until someone flipped a switch that woke me up with a blinding light.

I began reading and meditating for hours every day. My parents and friends thought I was going a bit crazy, but my life started improving rapidly. I was able to focus more clearly and stay calm in difficult situations. My grades went up; I started dating the most amazing and kindest girl in school; and I was accepted at a college I had never thought would take me.

I also began to feel a spiritual thirst. I wanted to meet other people who had similar experiences, but I didn't know how. So I started looking into the eyes of people on the street to see if there was a light behind them—a spark. For some reason, I thought I would be able to see in their eyes if they were asleep or awake. It wasn't until later that I heard the saying: "The eyes are the window to the soul." When I did, I immediately knew that what I had been looking for was the soul—the light—in people.

In my search for kindred spirits and more knowledge about life, I earned a degree in philosophy. I lived in ashrams in the Himalayas and traveled through East Asia. I studied with several gurus and spent seven years learning the mystic healing arts in Hawaii.

I did all this because, even after my initial awakening at sixteen, I still had so much to learn. I had to grow, to travel, to tap into my creativity. I had to experience heartbreak and loss. I had to build a career and slowly develop into a teacher. I had to learn who I really was, and how to live a truly meaningful life. In this way, my experience was similar to that of many spiritual seekers who came before me. Little did I know that these experiences would lead me to discover the seven archetypal energies that would bring my own soul into balance.

This book tells the story of my journey. In it, I explore each of these unique energies in balance, in deficit, and in excess. Using stories from my own life and those of my students, I examine the inherent challenges of each energy, as well as the consequences of their imbalance. Then I suggest specific tools and practices that can help you unlock the powers and gifts of each energy so you can begin to recognize that what you may see as "problems" in your life are actually opportunities to unleash the power of your soul.

We all embody all seven energies all the time, although many of us may feel particularly out of touch with one or more of them at any given moment. So, in addition to introducing and discussing these energies in depth, each chapter offers suggestions for how you can bring them into balance and apply them in your day-to-day life. My hope is that, when you understand your own soul energy through these seven archetypes, you will be able to find your own answers to life's challenges and questions.

The key, as you will discover here, is *balance*. Have you ever heard a choir sing? One person begins singing softly and beautifully, then another joins in, and then another. All of a sudden, the entire choir bursts into song and a harmonious, almost magical, sound emerges. That's how the seven energies of the soul work together in us when they are in balance. I hope this book will help you create that harmony on your own journey through life.

# Chapter 1

# Energy and Self-Realization

*The two most important days in your life are the day you are born and the day you find out why.*
—Mark Twain

Since the beginning of time, humans have sought out masters, oracles, and sages to find the meaning of life and answers to other deep questions. In ancient Greece, people walked hundreds of miles to the oracle at Delphi to be healed and to have their questions answered. In the time of the Buddha, groups of hundreds, sometimes thousands, of monks gathered to follow him across India, sitting and meditating, searching for answers to their deepest questions— searching for self-realization.

After forty-five years of traveling and teaching, as he was breathing his last breath, the Buddha told his followers: *Don't look to me for your answers; look inside yourself. I've given you the tools; now use them on yourself.*

Some listened. But most built statues to their teacher and formed different religious sects around his teachings. Then they began praying to him for their answers. Over the centuries, the Buddha became an object of worship to millions. Sound familiar? You could say the same things about Jesus, and about many other spiritual teachers as well.

The story usually goes like this. These teachers experience great suffering and retreat into a forest or a cave or climb a mountain. There, through self-reflection, they discover profound truths deep within themselves, which they then share with others. After departing their bodies, they ascend to the heavens and watch as their disciples misinterpret their teachings, fight among themselves, and fall back on dogma and ideology, reducing their teachings to a poor reflection of their original insights.

I admit that I have been guilty of playing this game myself. When I first went to India, I walked around with pictures of all my favorite gurus tucked into my pocket like baseball cards. I traveled from ashram to ashram, from guru to guru, listening to anyone with a beard, always believing that I would find someone else holding the key to my own self-realization. Think of how you feel when you open your high school yearbook and get a bit red in the face when you see what a dork you were. That's how

I feel sometimes when I think about how I used to idealize gurus.

I remember getting into a taxi in Thailand when I was at the beginning of my spiritual journey in my early twenties. The driver had one of those fat Buddha sculptures sitting on his dashboard. When I asked him about his connection to the Buddhist tradition, he rubbed the Buddha's belly and said: "Buddha brings me money." So much for my naive fantasy that all Buddhists were devout sages only interested in enlightenment!

Years later, as my understanding of the spiritual quest matured, I became the director of a school in Hawaii that taught mysticism. It was there that I began to find myself in a position similar to that of the teachers I had once followed. Referred by friends, people began to approach me to see if I could give them answers or heal their pain. One man even said: "I'd like you to give me an answer to a relationship question. I heard you can do some magic on me." To which I responded: "I can't do that, but I can teach you tools so you can find the answers within yourself." He gave me an irritated look and walked out. He wasn't ready to recognize that he was the only one who could find his own answers.

What I've come to realize over my years of helping people find their own answers is that the answers *always* lie within because they are born out of our own energy. I'll say it again: *All answers lie within because they are born out of our own energy.*

And that's a key word in this book—energy. So let me take a moment to explain what I mean by energy, because an understanding of *soul* energy is going to play a huge role in our journey together.

## Soul Energy

At a scientific level, energy is the force that moves all things. But in spiritual traditions, the term *energy* extends out beyond this basic definition to encompass the vital spark within your being that gives you life. This is the light I was looking for behind the eyes of those I passed on the street. This potent life force—this spiritual energy—operates within all of us. It animates and sustains us. It is our inner fire. It is what keeps us going through the inevitable difficulties and setbacks we all eventually face on our journeys. Religions and spiritual traditions around the world have different names for this energy—*prana, chi, pneuma, mana, baraka, shakti, vital force, nagual, wakan*, and of course, *spirit*. But for me personally, *soul* is the word that resonates the most. For me, your soul *is* the energy of your being. In my belief, soul and energy are the same thing.

But this belief presents a problem. Saying that your soul and energy are the same thing may sound great, but it is not really that helpful when it comes to navigating the world. Both the soul and energy are invisible and unquantifiable, which only adds to our difficulty in understanding their meaning. Although I knew from deep inside myself that we are made up of this powerful energy, and that accessing it was the key to leading a life of purpose and passion, I had a hard time articulating my belief to people in a way that was helpful.

And the need to do so was real. As I taught and counseled students over the course of ten years through the complicated and turbulent waters of life, I began to notice something remarkable. They were coming to me over and over with the same types of issues and struggles. The names, places, and situations were different, of course, but the core issues remained the same. When I talked to them about their energy—about the longings and needs of their souls that called out to be addressed—I could see that, while they may have understood the concepts on an intellectual level, they weren't absorbing them at a deeper level. It was all too nebulous.

And that's when something remarkable happened.

## The Seven Energy Archetypes

One day, in my own deep meditation, I was given an insight that I knew would help people understand the energy of the soul. In a moment of deep personal realization, I became aware of seven distinct energy archetypes, the names of which appeared spontaneously in my consciousness. These archetypes provide an accessible and powerful way for everyone to implement concrete change in their lives by balancing and harnessing their soul energy. I know this to be true, because I've seen it happen with my own students. In fact, these archetypes have proven to be the missing key for many of my students.

These are the seven energy archetypes that came to me in my meditation, along with their fundamental characteristics:

- **The Creator:** builder, maker, doer

- **The Healer:** sensitive, empathic, compassionate

- **The Warrior:** confident, disciplined, protective

- **The Lover:** nurturing, caring, romantic

- **The Artist:** expressive, original, imaginative

- **The Explorer:** curious, open-minded, courageous

- **The Master:** teaching, truth-seeking, introspective

I want to be clear that you don't possess or express only one or two of these energies. You aren't just an Artist or just a Healer. Your destiny in life is not defined by just one or two energies. Rather it is enriched and expanded by having access to all seven. Every one of us possesses *all of these energies in every moment*, in much the same way that white light contains all colors of the rainbow just waiting to be expressed through a prism.

At certain times, one energy may take center stage and become a dominant theme in your life. Then you may find your center of gravity shifting toward a different energy. You may even experience major shifts—like going from being a counselor, embodying your Healer archetype, to becoming a teacher, embodying your Master archetype.

You may also experience small shifts. You may even embody several energies, or even all seven energies, in a single day. You may embody the Lover when you make breakfast for your family, and later embody the Creator in your workplace. You may embody the Healer when a distressed friend calls you for help, and the Artist when you spend time writing in your journal or working on your guitar playing before bed.

While it is tempting to think of yourself as reflecting a single archetype most of the time—Artist, Healer, Warrior—the fact is that you can become any of them at any given moment simply by embracing and expressing that energy and its characteristics. On the basketball court or in the boardroom, you may be a Warrior. In the classroom, you may be a Master. On a mountaintop or in a laboratory, you may be an Explorer. And in each instance, you are fulfilling the potential of that energy in you.

Throughout this book you will learn how to find these transcendent energies in yourself and how to harness them in new ways. When you understand the detailed characteristics of each one, you will be able to shift your energy when you face an issue or challenge in a life associated with each archetype. In relationships, for example, there will undoubtedly be times when you need to access your Lover, your Healer, or even your Master energy. At work, you may need to be the Creator, Explorer, Artist, or Warrior.

As you deepen your understanding of each energy and become more practiced at how to shift and balance them, the truth of your soul will naturally begin to express itself to its fullest capacity. This feels like magic when it happens, but it is really just the natural consequence of working with your life through the lens of the seven energies. Through this work, you learn to uncover the purpose and passion in each area of your life like never before.

## Balancing the Energies

I used to be ashamed about feeling heartbreak and isolation after a few of my relationships ended badly. *I meditate all day long*, I thought. *I'm being honest and sharing my feelings*, I told myself. *Why am I still having such a hard time with intimate relationships?* Well, now I know that there wasn't anything wrong with me. I just needed to work with my Lover energy.

Although I had already worked to develop my inner Healer, Creator, and Master, the truth was that I hadn't really worked diligently on my inner Lover. And it needed attention, badly. Old pain from my formative years had left me out of balance and struggling in my relationships, and it wasn't until I admitted that to myself and worked on it specifically that I was able to form true bonds with others.

There's an important lesson in this: *It's often easier to see where others are out of balance in a specific energy than it is to see it in ourselves.*

I've seen many successful people feel confused when an underdeveloped part of their inner self starts pulling down the more refined parts. I've had clients who are CEOs of big corporations who can't understand intimate relationships. I've seen artists who are famous for their own work who can't grasp how to teach others the basics. I've known spiritual teachers who are great at delivering their message but are utterly lost when it comes to finances and business. So while we all have energies with which we are naturally aligned, if we allow the other energies of our souls to atrophy, ultimately these inner imbalances will drag down our entire experience. And that's why it's important to address them all and keep them in balance.

For example, you may have incredible potential to be a Healer in your community—to help people you know, to bridge divides in communication between loved ones, to help heal trauma. Yet for some reason, the Healer archetype just doesn't resonate with you. That may mean that, in order to activate your Healer potential, you must first heal yourself from your own past experiences that are still causing you emotional pain. Perhaps no one ever taught you how to do this, and so perhaps that Healer energy was never really activated in you. In this case, your Healer archetype may remain underdeveloped, and you may naturally feel out of touch with it because of this. In fact, it's often our own ideas about ourselves, the world, and our potential that stand in the way of our energies coming into balance.

In my own case, I love telling jokes and making people laugh. But I held an old belief that spiritual teachers weren't supposed to be funny; they were supposed to be serious. For years, I was afraid to unleash my inner comic because I didn't think I was supposed to be teaching meditation and making jokes at the same time. Then one day, it occurred to me that I just had to face the fact that my sense of humor was a part of me—an important part—and I wouldn't be teaching anything as my full authentic self until I made humor a part of my work.

Soon after, I started joking in my meditations. I got a lot of great feedback from people who enjoyed my teachings more because they were not so serious. Suddenly, I was helping more people than ever before, especially those who had struggled with meditation and had put so much pressure on themselves to do it perfectly.

Including humor in my guided meditations helped put my students at ease and allowed them to step away from their own old ideas about the "seriousness" of meditation and spiritual growth. True, I also got some criticism from some, but they were definitely in the minority. Overall, I felt as if I were being true to myself, connecting to my students as the real me. And the result was that I was reaching more people than ever before. The comic in me is part of my Artist energy. And until that part of me started to flower, it was holding back my growth as a meditation teacher, which was part of my Master energy.

My point is that these energies are not isolated forces. They are not separate from one another. They cross over; they balance each other; they depend on each other. They complement each other like the legs of a table. They are like the separate parts of the body. The heart needs the brain, the brain needs the nervous system, and so on. They all work together.

As you recognize which of your energies need work and focus on bringing them into balance, it may feel almost like finding a hidden spiritual power that has been lying dormant within you. Don't be surprised if the world begins to shift around you in new and fascinating ways. Magical things happen when we access these energies and work with them in a way that aligns with our deepest truth. This is something that I want for each and every person on this planet.

## Energy Inventory

We will go into the seven energies in detail in the chapters to come, but before we do so, I want you to look at the list of the seven energy archetypes and consider your first reaction to each. In the exercise below, indicate, on a scale of 1 to 10, whether it is an energy with which you naturally identify or one to which you don't feel as connected. We will come back to this exercise as we progress through the book.

---

**THE CREATOR: BUILDER, MAKER, DOER**

No Connection . . . . . . . . Some Connection . . . . . . . . Strong Connection

1_____2_____3_____4_____5_____6_____7_____8_____9_____10

---

**THE HEALER: SENSITIVE, EMPATHIC, COMPASSIONATE**

No Connection . . . . . . . . Some Connection . . . . . . . . Strong Connection

1_____2_____3_____4_____5_____6_____7_____8_____9_____10

---

**THE WARRIOR: CONFIDENT, DISCIPLINED, PROTECTIVE**

No Connection . . . . . . . . Some Connection . . . . . . . . Strong Connection

1_____2_____3_____4_____5_____6_____7_____8_____9_____10

## THE LOVER: NURTURING, CARING, ROMANTIC

No Connection . . . . . . . . Some Connection . . . . . . . . Strong Connection

1____2____3____4____5____6____7____8____9____10

## THE ARTIST: EXPRESSIVE, ORIGINAL, IMAGINATIVE

No Connection . . . . . . . . Some Connection . . . . . . . . Strong Connection

1____2____3____4____5____6____7____8____9____10

## THE EXPLORER: CURIOUS, OPEN-MINDED, COURAGEOUS

No Connection . . . . . . . . Some Connection . . . . . . . . Strong Connection

1____2____3____4____5____6____7____8____9____10

## THE MASTER: TEACHING, TRUTH-SEEKING, INTROSPECTIVE

No Connection . . . . . . . . Some Connection . . . . . . . . Strong Connection

1____2____3____4____5____6____7____8____9____10

Chapter 2

# The Pursuit of Balance

*Your hand opens and closes, opens and closes. If
it were always a fist or always stretched open, you
would be paralysed. Your deepest presence is in
every small contracting and expanding, the two as
beautifully balanced and coordinated as birds' wings.*

—Jelaluddin Rumi

I once had a client who was the CEO of a thriving
company. He was extremely well paid and enjoyed a
generous expense account, stock options, and other
perks. He lived in a big house in an exclusive neigh-
borhood, drove a fancy car, and traveled extensively.
By all current cultural standards, he was a highly successful person.

But he had a problem. He absolutely hated his job.

It hadn't always been that way, of course. When he
first started with the company, he liked the industry
and enjoyed what he did, and that was largely why he

had been so successful. But now, twenty years later, he dreaded going to work every day. His likes and interests had changed, and he didn't know what to do.

After we did some initial exploratory work together (using self-reflection practices I include later in this book), he uncovered several important revelations. He learned that his job didn't align with what he really wanted for himself now and in the next phase of his life. And this lack of alignment was causing a lot of pain for him and for the people closest to him. Even so, he was resistant to making any real changes based on these realizations, because he feared that doing so might mean that he would no longer be "successful." He was afraid to give up the image that he'd built of himself.

Then he suddenly found himself grappling with a series of business-related problems, one right after the other—customer lawsuits, investor revolts, financial stress. It was as if the universe had decided to shift the ground beneath his feet in order to push him to make changes.

Perhaps you've experienced a time in your own life when things shifted in an unexpected way that was painful at first, but ultimately proved to be necessary and constructive. Of course, it's often much easier to see this kind of shift as beneficial in hindsight, and that turned out to be the case for my client.

I could tell in our early visits that he was struggling to accept the setbacks. Despite what I said, he insisted on attacking them head-on with all his Warrior and Creator abilities, determined to fix each and every one. He hired high-priced lawyers, worked eighty-hour weeks, and tried everything in his power to force events in the direction he thought they should go. Ultimately, however, this kind of struggle can't last forever.

After several months of battle, he finally decided to surrender the fight. This meant that he had to let go of his old ideas about who he was and where he was "supposed to be" in his life and career. When he was forced out of his job by the board of directors, he actually felt an enormous sense of relief. And it wasn't long before he was offered a position that was more aligned with his new passions. I'm happy to report that he is far happier and more fulfilled now than he had been for the last several years at his old job.

There are a couple of important lessons in this man's story.

## Excess and Deficiency

When things first started to go wrong for him, this CEO's initial response was to double down on his Creator and Warrior archetypes by fighting against the shifting landscape beneath his feet. These energies came very easily to him; he was more naturally attuned to them than he was to some of the other energies. But unfortunately, he was applying these energies *in the wrong direction.* He was relying on what I refer to as "energy in excess." We all have the potential to do this, because it is natural for us to fall back on the energy with which we feel most aligned.

You may know (or be) someone who has excess Creator energy. We often call them workaholics, as they are obsessed with creating and producing, often at the expense of family time and leisure. Likewise, those with excess Warrior energy tend to become hypercompetitive, unable to lose at anything gracefully, even something as seemingly trivial as a board game with friends.

So while it is important that we develop the energies we feel are deficient within us, it's equally important to be aware of those energies we may have in excess. This is where the exercise you did at the end of chapter 1 can provide some insight. It's often the energies with which we feel naturally aligned that can become developed to excess. And this throws us out of energetic balance.

As you will soon see, the good life is *all about balance.* The key to a happy and fulfilling life lies in the balance of the seven energies. It may seem easier to work on developing the energies you see as deficient.

Most of us are programmed to do that. But it's harder to see when an excess of a certain energy is impacting us negatively. We will look at the consequences of deficiency and excess in each of the seven energies in the following chapters.

## Defining Success

The next lesson we can glean from this man's story is how important it is to acknowledge and honor our own definition of success. The definition my client found himself trapped in is perhaps the most common one in our current cultural climate. From the moment we're born, we are inundated with messages from society that success means finding the highest-paying job available and then working ourselves to the bone achieving as much money, status, power, and material goods as we can. This picture may shift a bit depending on your own personal upbringing, but, for most of us, the message is that "success" is dependent on acquisition, achievement, accumulation, and attainment. If personal happiness or self-fulfillment are mentioned at all, they are considered as prizes or rewards that can only be won as a result of these achievements.

So before we go any further in this book, I want to share with you my own definition of success. Success for me is living a life of passion and purpose. It's a life in which, on most days, I feel happy and fulfilled. It's a life in which I march to the beat of my own drum.

Because we are all unique, this passionate and purposeful life will be different for each and every one of us. But the common theme in them all is *balance*. It is through balancing the seven energies that we can bring passion and purpose to our lives. As we move through each energy in the chapters that follow, my hope is that you'll learn to recognize what true success looks like for you. I am often asked by clients whether learning to balance the seven energies of the soul will bring them lots of money, or a big house, or the perfect partner. The answer of course is no, it won't automatically cause those things to happen. It is possible that they *may* happen as a natural consequence to becoming your whole self, but these kinds of achievements are not the goal. True success is the outward expression of inner balance.

When we find energetic balance, we find a joy and fulfillment in life that can't be found in any other way. Once you become familiar with the seven energies and how they manifest in your life, you will be able to look within anytime you feel "off," and see which of the energies needs to be brought into balance.

A student once approached the Buddha, upset about how his meditation practice was going.

"What happens when you string an instrument too tightly?" the Buddha asked him.

"The string breaks."

"And what happens when you string it too loosely?"

"No sound comes out," the student answered. "To produce a tuneful sound, the strings must be neither too tight or too loose."

"And that," the Buddha replied, "is how to practice. Not too tight, not too loose."

Success is balance. Happiness is born out of balance. When the seven energies are functioning properly together in a balanced way, this balance leads to a life of purpose and fulfillment. In my experience, the answer to every problem we experience is within us. Knowing how to find and access the right energy can lead us to our inner answers sooner and with less suffering.

In the following chapters, I give you four tools that can help you find that balance—meditation, self-reflection, setting goals, and taking action. Let's take some time now to look at each of these practices before we dive in.

## Meditation

Meditation can be intimidating because traditional descriptions of the practice still tend to emphasize specific postures that can be difficult for some. Other descriptions seem to imply that a "quiet mind" is the same as experiencing no thoughts in the mind at all. Of course, neither of these is true. Sitting for meditation can be as simple as sitting up straight in a chair, and every person who meditates struggles with the chatter of the mind. But achieving some false notion of perfection in meditation is not the goal; *meditating*—pursuing stillness and accepting who you are in this moment—is a goal in and of itself.

The benefits of meditation that you hear about so often in the media come from regular practice. When you set an intention to meditate regularly, you are essentially making a date with your inner self. When you continually show up for that date, your inner self will respond by revealing your potential to tap into your own depths and achieve peace. It's that simple.

On a practical level, you don't need to set aside some dedicated space or room in your house for this. Of course, if you wish to and have the space, please feel free. All you really need to do, however, is to find a position in which you can sit comfortably without falling asleep for at least twenty to thirty minutes. You may prefer to sit on the ground with your legs crossed, or on a cushion (there are many cushions that are especially designed for meditation), or in a chair. The important thing to remember is that, in all instances, your back should be straight and you should try not to lean against anything (though you can use a back rest if needed). Your head should rest lightly on the top of your spine. Your hands can sit gently in your lap. If you are familiar with particular hand positions (called *mudras* in Eastern traditions) and feel they help you, definitely use them, but this is not necessary. Nor is sitting in what is commonly referred to as "the lotus position," something that may be particularly difficult for those with knee issues. This is not an exercise in pain tolerance! Whatever position helps you to maintain a state of *relaxed alertness,* that is the best position for you.

In each of the following chapters, I give a meditation exercise that focuses on coming back into balance within the context of the target energy. I have also created a free downloadable audio meditation for each of the energies that can be found on my website: www.meditationschool.us. If you want to go more deeply into any deficiencies or excesses you feel in an energy, you can find bonus meditations on my site as well.

## Self-Reflection

One of the main benefits of meditation is that it opens up a space in which we can engage in some deep discovery about ourselves. While I am a big fan of meditation and its many benefits, there are those in the meditation community who think they can meditate their way through any problem. In most cases, however, this simply isn't true.

When we combine meditation with powerful inner exploration and self-reflection, however, we really start to see results. When we examine our ideas, beliefs, and any past experiences that have caused us suffering—when we make a commitment to undo, or change, or forgive, or accept what we find—we can make lasting changes in our lives.

To help you develop a sound practice of self-reflection, I've included a series of exploratory questions at the end of each chapter. These are meant only as a jumping-off point for your own reflection, so feel free to go beyond them to wherever your own personal needs may lead you. I recommend that you engage with these questions in writing, in a journal or notebook. There's a special magic that happens when you write things down, as you can see them more clearly and notice patterns in yourself that you might not have noticed otherwise.

Keeping everything inside your head is often part of the problem, as our thoughts can become so jumbled and overwhelming that we get lost in them. By recording your thoughts in a journal that is for your eyes only, you can reflect on them without any inhibition or judgment—except of course, your own, which is, after all, your goal. To be clear, your journal certainly doesn't need to be anything fancy, but you may wish to purchase a special book just for this purpose.

## Setting Goals and Taking Action

Our word-focused, online culture makes it easy to spend all of our time in our heads. Of course, reading, thinking, and discerning *are* critical. And meditation and self-reflection are powerful tools. But we can get lost in them. Eventually, you must set a goal and take action in order to go beyond thinking and bring the lessons of the seven energies into your physical body and the world at large.

Ultimately, our goal in working with these energies is to manifest balance in every aspect of our daily lives, whether that's sitting with a cup of hot tea and our private thoughts in the morning, taking the subway to work surrounded by the incredible diversity of our fellow human beings, or hiking through a river valley and marveling at the plants and animals that live there. We want to find peace in it all.

At the end of each of the following chapters, I suggest some goals you can set and some actions you can take to help bring balance to each energy in your life. These are relatively easy practices that are simple to implement, like trying something new or taking a walk in nature. But just because they are simple and easy, don't let your mind convince you that they aren't necessary.

## Three Essential Attitudes

The seven energies are always with us, and our work with them allows us to move with more grace and confidence through all the situations we come across in our lives. Through balancing them properly, we uncover the power of true success and learn how to avoid the pitfalls of excess and deficiency. But before we begin our examination of each energy, there are three essential attitudes I want you to take with you as you move forward. They are radical self-honesty, self-acceptance, and self-compassion.

### Radical Self-Honesty

The fastest way to work through a block or come to a realization is to be uncompromisingly honest about what you feel and what you experience when you close your eyes to meditate and when you answer the self-reflection questions at the end of each chapter. I encourage you to refrain from manipulating how you feel or trying to think your way around resistance. Just be honest with yourself. These practices are for your eyes only, so don't be afraid to acknowledge your true feelings. If you experience sadness, be sad. If you're angry, let the anger work itself out. If you invalidated, or unworthy, let that energy hav in the sun so it doesn't linger in your unconsciou manipulate you from the shadows.

Being truly honest with yourself and how you feel is the first, and most important, step toward balance.

### Self-Acceptance

Sometimes, after we are really honest with ourselves, we immediately start to judge ourselves: *I can't believe I feel this way. This is proof I am a horrible person!* This is 100 percent untrue! One of the things you can learn from meditation is that your thoughts are largely beyond your control, and they often arise from your social conditioning. Remember: Thoughts are just thoughts; they aren't "real" in the world. They only exist in your mind and, just because you have them, doesn't mean you will act on them.

The Buddhist tradition sees thoughts as metaphoric clouds in the sky of awareness. But imagine the sky being upset with the shape of a cloud, and then judging it as bad. We quickly recognize this as silly. Yet most of us tend to do this with our own thoughts (if we are being radically honest with ourselves). I want you to accept yourself exactly as you are, and this means spotting and releasing any self-judgment that arises. Those judgments are the sticky substance that allows negative emotions to cling to you. Self-acceptance is what allows you to peel them away, slowly and gently.

### Self-Compassion

The balm of self-compassion is the key to transforming "problems" into opportunities that serve a purpose. Compassion is acceptance with love and understanding woven into it. It's much easier for most people to have compassion for others, however, than it is for them to have it for themselves. But that's because we are in a constant race to be better. Most likely, you've been through a lot in your life and it hasn't always been easy. If it had been, you probably wouldn't be reading this book.

You must learn to show yourself some respect and love when you come upon pain, sadness, pockets of self-judgment, a noisy mind, or self-defeating beliefs. Through self-compassion, you learn, not only to accept yourself, but to know that you are worthy to be cared for and loved.

## Back to Balance

Based on the exercise we did at the end of chapter 1, you may already have an intuitive sense of the energies that are either deficient or excessive in your life. These are the energies that you need to work on personally. You may also have a sense of the energies in which you feel confident and balanced. Naturally, you may be drawn to the chapters that treat those energies first. While there is certainly no right or wrong way to use this book, I do recommend that you read the detailed description of each energy to give yourself a greater understanding of how each one manifests in your life. You may be surprised to find some deficiency or excess you didn't previously suspect. Moreover, having a clear understanding of each energy will help you deal with future challenges. Most of us experience deficiency and excess in different energies at different times in our lives. That's just how the universe works!

### Meditation to Begin Our Journey

We're just about ready to dive into the seven energies in detail, but here, at the very beginning of our journey, let's take a few moments to prepare with a short meditation.

> **Step 1:** Set the stage for seeing clearly by placing your index fingers on your temples, one on each side of your head. If you feel the need to do so, massage your temples for a moment. Notice that, between your physical temples, lies your "mental temple." This is

where most of your consciousness happens—in the center of your head.

**Step 2:** Close your eyes and imagine that the center of your head is a room. The lights are on; there is a floor, perhaps a hardwood floor or a carpet. There may be some furniture or a few familiar items. In the center of this room, there is a seat, a chair, or a cushion.

**Step 3:** Sit down in this place in the center of your head and look out in front of you, where there is a projector screen you can use to view various memories and images. Create and project an image of an orange onto that screen. See it floating out in front of you. Notice the color, the shape, the texture. Then watch it explode like fireworks and turn to dust.

**Step 4:** Next, try an image of a sunflower. A beautiful yellow sunflower. Notice its petals, its shape, the details of its stem. Take a moment to appreciate the image, and then let it go. Send it off into the stars and watch it disappear in the sky. If you feel as if you can't see anything, imagine what something might look like if you *could* see it. What if you imagined a sunflower? Do your best, but don't strain yourself.

**Step 5:** Now call up a recent memory of a time when you had some fun. See it as an image on the screen of your mind. Make sure it's far enough away so that you aren't pushed right up against it, but not so far away that you can't make out the details. Perhaps the image even sits in a picture frame.

**Step 6:** Notice the borders of the image. Then notice the energy or the feeling quality of the memory. Is it happy? Expansive? Dense? Heavy? Confusing? Inspiring? See that it has its own energy that animates it. And notice that, if you lose yourself in the image, you may start feeling the emotions of the memory in your body and get lost in them.

**Step 7:** Back out of the image, smile, and let it go. Turn it to dust.

Now let's explore the seven energy archetypes together.

Chapter 3

# The Creator

*A rock pile ceases to be a rock pile the moment a single man contemplates it, bearing within him the image of a cathedral.*
—Antoine de Saint-Exupéry

Humans are fundamentally creative beings. From the very beginning of our time here on this planet, we have built civilizations filled with astonishing architecture, invented increasingly complex machinery and technology, advanced the art of medicine and healing, and developed systems of production and exchange that have moved us beyond the need to hunt, or gather, or grow our own food—although there is something to be said for doing so. We are innately curious. We want to know: *How? Why? What if . . .?* Answering those questions has left behind a millennia-long legacy of human innovation. We are makers and doers. And this remarkable ability—this potent energy—exists within every single one of us.

To be human is to create. Creativity is in our DNA; it is our birthright.

At its core, Creator energy is the essence in you that manifests as the desire to do, to make, to build, to grow, or to invent. The Creator wants to take an idea or concept and give it life. Creator energy gives physical form to the human spirit. It is the connection between the soul and the world—the intangible and tangible. It fulfills us by moving energy from the dimension of potential to the realm of matter. Creators generate ideas and beliefs, but also value getting things done.

## The Creator in Balance

Many people hear the word *creative* and automatically think of the arts. For our purposes, however, these two energies—Artist and Creator—while often working in tandem, encompass different strengths. We'll explore the Artist in chapter 7; here, we'll focus on the Creator as inventor and builder. In Creator energy, we find the innate desire and ability to *manifest*—to take an idea and translate it into reality.

This is the part of you that wakes up in the middle of the night with an idea that you can't seem to stop thinking about. It's that part of you that opens a computer document or a journal page to start writing down a plan.

The Creator in you may be interested in anything from building a business, to creating a new technology, to starting or growing a family, to building literal buildings, to developing any kind of practical solution to a problem or need. Creators also know that, through creation and iteration, slowly but surely, things become more and more useful, innovative, and beautiful. To them, it's not about achieving perfection, but about the joy of inventing, of molding, of building.

Those with balanced Creator energy are:

- Grounded

- Practical

- Active

- Inventive

- Direct

- Energetic

- Problem-solvers

- Hardworking

- Entrepreneurial

- Innovative

Creator energy is often, but not exclusively, connected to our careers—making money, finding stability, and achieving our life goals in some way. And achieving some of these goals may require that we see something that doesn't yet exist. In fact, without visualization, the Creator in you may begin to feel blind or lost on your path. A healthy Creator sees an image in the mind's eye, sees a problem being solved, sees something beyond the horizon—and *commits to taking action*.

One of the biggest ironies is that, despite the fact that all humans are clearly creative, many don't see themselves that way. We often hear people say things like: "I'm not creative," or "I could never do something like that." In fact, for a long time, I didn't think I was a Creator. I thought Creators had to look like my father, who designed skyscrapers in New York City. Although I hadn't developed the concept of Creator energy then, I grew up believing that a Creator was someone who only built tangible objects like buildings.

Those beliefs created limitations in me. But as I developed into a meditation teacher and built a living around my own unique skill set, I began to realize that building my coaching practice required that I use a form of Creator energy as well. When I found myself managing people who worked for me, working with meditation apps, leading retreats, and creating my online meditation school, I realized that I was tapping into my Creator energy. I was just doing it in a different way than the adults I had observed when I was growing up.

To be a healthy Creator, it's important to honor yourself as such. You must tether your vision to your values, and learn to pull on that thin intuitive thread that will lead you in the right direction. The exercises at the end of this chapter will help you do that. And remember, how you create may be totally different from how others that you respect or consider Creators do.

## The Creator in Deficit

We all have Creator energy inside us. But sometimes we have trouble tapping into it. We may find ourselves feeling small, lost, or invalidated when we begin to make something. Or we may be afraid of sharing our ideas or inventions with the world. We may be hesitant to take risks or to let others see our potential imperfections. If we stay in this pattern long enough, we may even form an identity around it: *I have ideas but never follow through.* And this can become a self-fulfilling prophecy. The irony is that we may become subconsciously afraid of succeeding, because, if we do, we lose the very identity we created!

Deficient Creator energy manifests as:

- Apathy

- Unwillingness to try new things

- Fear of being seen

- A debilitating fear of failure

- Difficulty finishing projects

- Giving in to feelings of invalidation

- Inaction due to a need to be perfect

- Making unhealthy comparisons to others

- A lack of self-confidence

- Self-judgment

- A belief that everything has already been thought of

- Lack of self-worth

But the good news is that all of these fears can be overcome once you become aware of them. Barriers to activating your Creator energy include a tendency to make unhealthy comparisons, a fear of failure, the need to be perfect, and what I call "not-enoughism."

### Unhealthy Comparisons

One of the first barriers to Creator energy is erected when we compare ourselves to others. In fact, there are few things that can stop Creator energy in its tracks as effectively as this. For instance, when I was getting ready to create my first online meditation video, I was standing on a small stepladder putting up a green screen when I had this very clear thought: *I'll never be as good as my own teacher—he has so much wisdom, charisma, and presence.* It was so clear that I could even see it in a specific area of my mind.

At that moment, I actually fell off the ladder and hit my head—in the exact place I'd seen the thought! Lying on the floor, I wanted to quit right then and there. I was stuck fast in my own feelings of not being "good enough." But luckily, I didn't quit. Instead, I eventually recognized that I was sabotaging myself by making these comparisons. I realized that comparison is actually a death knell for Creator energy—nothing squelches it faster.

In reality, the other teacher was doing his thing, and I was doing mine. Comparing myself to him was zapping my own Creator energy around my project, so I had to let it go. And I did. What I learned is that, in moments like these, just recognizing or becoming aware that making comparisons can destroy your Creator energy is often enough to help you let those comparisons go. Ironically, just a few years later, that same teacher actually called me for business advice, wanting to know how I was creating all those great videos and how I had done such a good job of building a business around my passion!

### Fear of Failure

Another barrier to tapping into our Creator energy arises from our belief that past performance predicts future results. When we look to the past and see where we've tried before and "failed," we often see this as proof that we won't or can't succeed in the future. When we get caught in this loop of invalidation, we destroy our Creator energy.

An old adage tells us that good judgment comes from experience, and experience comes from poor judgment. When we avoid failure, we deny ourselves the feedback we need to become successful. Instead of seeing our past efforts as "failures," we must see them as a way to gain experience and find out what doesn't work. Thus our "failures" become instrumental in building our success.

The first rocket ever built never made it into space, and the first loaf of bread ever baked was probably not delicious. Intellectually, we all know this. But if we focus on our "failures" and beat ourselves up over them, we further alienate ourselves from our

Creator energy. Imagine if the first rocket scientists had dwelled on their initial attempts. They would have blocked their Creator energy so completely that they never would have made it off the launchpad.

### The Need to be Perfect

This barrier to Creator energy is harder to spot, because it pretends to be an asset. I'm talking about perfectionism—the need to get everything right (and right the first time), to never make mistakes, to never be seen as anything less than flawless. We're often told by society that we should constantly aim for this transcendent state of sheer perfection. But the truth is that this obsession with being perfect can actually prevent us from stepping up to the starting line in the first place. Perfectionism is, in fact, an enemy of true creativity.

Perfectionism is born chiefly out of the very natural fear of rejection. We can all think of times when we were younger and felt the awful sensation of being rejected—whether perceived or real, whether from adults or from our peers, or even from societal messaging. As adults, we think we've moved past caring what other people think of us. But much of the time, this is belied by our relentless pursuit of perfection that stems from this buried fear. Author and researcher Brené Brown calls perfectionism a self-destructive and addictive belief system that fuels this primary thought: *If I look perfect, and do everything perfectly, I can avoid or minimize the painful feelings of shame, judgment, and blame.*

And this is how perfectionism becomes the enemy of true creativity. If creativity depends on the commitment to try new things despite the risk of failure—whether for the first or maybe even the 700th time—and perfectionism insists on protecting us from the shame and rejection we may feel when we fail, those afflicted by the need to be perfect may choose not to try anything new at all. And that's when Creator energy dwindles and wanes down to the merest whisper of what it could be.

### *"Not-Enoughism"*

Deep-seated beliefs that we are "not enough" comprise the most formidable barriers to Creator energy. The media bombards us daily with the message that, if we are not "enough"—pretty enough, smart enough, spiritual enough, strong enough—we will never find a romantic partner, fulfill our dreams, or achieve our goals. I can't tell you how many people I've counseled and coached who stalled their creative efforts out of a belief that they weren't ready or good enough.

This "not enoughism" is a form of constant societal rejection that we readily adopt and then believe to be true. In turn, this then provides fertile ground for perfectionism to grow. It's all interrelated, and guaranteed to create a deficiency in your Creator energy.

## The Creator in Excess

As I mentioned previously, we tend to focus on deficiencies when considering energy, but it's equally important to look at the other side of the issue—the problems that an excess of each energy can cause. Let's explore a bit about what that means when it comes to Creator energy.

Excessive Creator energy manifests as:

• Workaholism

• An inflated sense of self

• The need to prove ourselves

• Scattered energy

• Starting too many projects at once

• Selfishness

• Greed

• Obsession with success

- Forgetting what's truly important

- Constantly needing to solve problems

- Sacrificing relationships for work

When Creators in excess look deeply inside themselves, they may find a belief that their value as human beings is based on what they have created or need to create. Their net worth, their legacy, their status, or their material possessions may define them. Unreasonable goals may haunt them and push them into overdrive. In excess, Creators may look very successful from the outside, but struggle with low self-esteem on the inside.

Traits that can contribute to excessive Creator energy include an obsession with success, lack of focus, and avoiding personal needs.

### Obsession with Success

We've all seen CEOs who can't take a day off from work and neglect their families. Or entrepreneurs who believe they can fix the entire world with their enterprise. Or social media stars whose entire identity is based on their number of followers.

It may look easy—and it may even *be* easy for a time—for Creators in excess to appear successful in the eyes of the world. But when you inspect their lives more closely, you may find that they have a lot of unfulfilled relationships because they're too busy building and working all the time.

### Lack of Focus

Excess Creator energy can also stem from a desire to do too many things all at once. Creators in excess may have countless projects going, too many commitments new ideas being downloaded every moment, and they can't seem to manage it all. Their energy becomes unfocused and scattered. They may feel overwhelmed, or that there is not enough time in the day. They may fall prey to anxiety and stress from the pressure to complete or achieve something. This can leave them feeling ungrounded and trapped in a loop of frustration.

### Avoiding Personal Needs

I had a client once who asked me to work with her on her career. She was very successful in the tech industry and had reached a high level of achievement and status, but she kept getting caught up in drama and problems at work and it was making her miserable.

As we peeled back some of the layers in our sessions together, I could tell that she was a workaholic—something she proudly admitted. I suspected that part of the reason she was overworking was to avoid something in her personal life, which is often the case with workaholics. So I asked her how her love life was going, and she admitted that she had been avoiding dealing with her deep desire for a partner by overworking. In doing so, she was ignoring her heart. Her feelings of loneliness and unfulfillment eventually started spilling over into her work, manifesting in all sorts of strange and unnecessary dramas. She began unconsciously taking her resentment and anger out on her coworkers, and often felt like a victim. Her excess Creator energy was trying to make up for a deficiency in her Lover energy.

From this woman's perspective, her career and her love life were unrelated. But when she slowed down, she was able to recognize that the unhappiness from her unfulfilled relationship space was bleeding over into her work, causing chaos. When she admitted what she was missing in life and stopped avoiding the pain of it, she was able to start making space for a new relationship.

This is a great example of how the loss of balance can have serious negative repercussions in our lives.

## Back to Balance

Now let's focus on how to balance Creator energy and how to manifest it in our lives in authentic ways. Let me first say that it's easy for those who seek growth to focus on the negative in themselves and to try to fix every part of who they are. But we can easily get addicted to *fixing* ourselves.

To balance the Creator in ourselves, or any energy for that matter, we must stop trying to "fix" ourselves and begin to focus on what we want to create, so that we can reverse engineer it with confidence. To accomplish this, we need to tap into what we want to create at a very deep and authentic level. Then we have to learn how to visualize.

Remember: Creator energy is all about action. It's not enough to think about creating something or doing something. You have to commit to visualizing the stages of completion and then take action. Some have a hard time visualizing what they want; some even have a hard time actually *doing* what they want. But balanced Creator energy requires both to be successful. And you have the capacity for both. You just have to own it.

You don't need to inflate or deflate your sense of self to get what you want. Nor do you have to manipulate others. You don't have to spin endlessly in the waters of deficiency or excess, constantly trying to control, to perfect, or to fix yourself. You just need to be honest with yourself (radically honest) and to own the power of your Creator energy. Then you can use the fuel of your desires to see your next step in life and manifest that energy in action.

Here are some practices that can help you do that.

### Meditation to Balance Creator Energy

You can take as long as you need for this meditation; there is no correct amount of time. You'll probably need a minimum of fifteen minutes, however, to get deep into the meditation.

**Step 1:** As you close your eyes and draw your attention into the center of your head, notice you are sitting in a chair in a calm room. In front of you, visualize a well-used desk in a style that appeals to you. On top of the desk is a book called *The Creator* with your name listed as the author.

**Step 2:** As you flip open the book, you randomly turn to a page that is blank. As you touch this page, an image starts to form. This image represents a true calling of your inner Creator in action. It shows what you're ready to begin or finish building in your life.

**Step 3:** Take your time and study the image. If it's blurry, check to see if you're too close to it or too far away, as if you were reading words on a page and needed to focus your eyes at the right distance.

**Step 4:** What is it about this image that makes it special to you? What physical, emotional, mental, or spiritual need does it fulfill in your life?

**Step 5:** Can you own that this image belongs to you and represents a clear goal that you are here to achieve in this life? Can you feel that the Creator in you is here to manifest this image into form? Can you have confidence that this image is something you can create?

**Step 6:** Ask yourself what physical actions you need to take in order to engineer this image into reality. Are you willing to take these actions? Are you committed to taking these actions?

**Step 7:** Allow a color to glow around this image—any color that you feel best represents your current Creator energy. You may even feel it in your body. When you're ready, write a date at the top right of the blank page.

Feel the truth of this image as being part of your destiny as a Creator. Slowly close the book, sit back comfortably in your chair, and open your eyes.

Spend about ten minutes writing in your journal, noting every Creator project you want to do. As you work through the chapters in this book and look at your other energy patterns, you may want to revisit this list. How will you harness your energies to make these things happen?

### Creator Self-Reflection

Remember that meditation, while critical, is just one step in our work together. Try spending some time with the questions below and writing your responses in your journal to gain a comprehensive understanding of the state of your Creator energy. As you work through this book, try to spend at least a few days with each energy, considering these questions in depth.

Ask yourself these questions to determine if you have any deficient Creator tendencies:

- Do you avoid starting or finishing a project out of fear or apathy?

- Does your inner critic feel out of control when you create?

- Do you expend a lot of mental energy comparing your work to that of others?

- Do you avoid letting other people see your creations?

Now ask yourself these questions to determine if you have any excessive Creator tendencies:

- Do you overwork to avoid emotion or pain?

- Do you value your projects or work above all else?

- Do you think what you create or your success makes you special or better than others?

- Do you forget what's truly important in life because you are obsessed with your creations?

Finally, ask yourself these questions as you work to cultivate balanced Creator energy:

- If I had the time, energy, skill, and confidence, where would my Creator energy truly want to focus? What would it want to do or make in the world now?

- What deep need would manifesting this creation fulfill in my soul?

- Where in my life have I avoided owning my Creator energy?

- Where in my life has my Creator energy been in excess?

- Who in my life has a Creator energy that I admire and why?

- As my Creator energy rises to its full potential, how do I want to share it with the world?

- What is my next step toward truly living in my Creator energy?

### Creator Goals

Consider the difference between how Creator energy works internally and externally. Then see if you can come up with three ways in which you can apply your Creator energy to your life on an internal level. For example:

- Have more confidence in my ability to create wealth.

- Be more practical and grounded.

- Find something of value inside of me to offer the world.

Now write down three ways in which you can apply your Creator energy to your life on an external level. For example:

- Have a secure and grounded home.

- Build my website or business.

- Create my own online meditation school.

### Creator Action: A Date with Failure

If you've identified some Creator deficiencies in yourself, know that some of these may actually be the key to your ultimate success if you're willing to work through them. Of course, if you've identified primarily an excess of Creator energy in your life, you may want to move on to a different energy in which you are deficient first. But the activities in each chapter and in each energy are all designed to help you establish true balance, so don't worry that exercising an energy in which you are already in excess may push you further out of balance. The truth is that, once you recognize and begin to work with each of these energies in a conscious way, they will start to balance themselves naturally. And you can always come back to any of these meditations, questions, and exercises to work on different aspects of each energy.

As we explored above, the need to be perfect, "not-enoughism," and fear of failure and rejection are all tied together—so much so that we can actually find ourselves paralyzed by our fears and unable to take the first step toward trying anything new or risky. Our dreams are precious to us, and sometimes it can be overwhelming to think about all the ways in which they might not work out. But these failures are an unavoidable and critical part of the work. In fact, it's almost impossible to achieve your goals and dreams without failure. So why not build up your "failure" muscles (and subsequently your Creator energy) by exercising them in a conscious way that is not only fun, but also has slightly lower stakes. Become a "failure pro" when it comes to tackling your dreams.

For this exercise, first make a list of things you've always been interested in trying, but just haven't gotten around to yet or have avoided out of a "certainty" that you will be bad at them. These can be as small or as grand as you like—for example: playing a musical instrument, learning to cook or bake (or trying particularly challenging recipes), writing a sonnet, drawing a portrait, sewing a piece of clothing, building a piece of furniture, throwing a pot on a potter's wheel, or organizing a small event in your area. Choose one item from your list, then commit to trying it out for at least one month.

The actual activity you choose is secondary to the work here. You may even find that, after the month is over, you don't want to continue with it because it's "not your thing." And that's fine. The point is not necessarily to master a new hobby or activity. The point is to train yourself to accept and even welcome failure. Of course, you will be bad at any new skill at first. Violin virtuosos made the same horrible scratchy ear-piercing noises when they first picked up the instrument as you will. Soufflés fall. Early drawings look weird and out of proportion. The amazing people who spring to mind when you think of the best of the best in any area started at the beginning just like you. And then they failed—over and over again—until they got better at it. And the better they got, the more they realized that their failures were actually their best teachers.

# Chapter 4

# The Healer

*We cannot heal what we cannot feel.*
—John Bradshaw

The next essential energy of the soul is one with which many emotionally sensitive people identify: the Healer. The Healer yearns to take things that are separate or broken and make them whole and complete. This energy fulfills its purpose by helping people reduce pain, find resolution to conflict, mend broken parts, or heal trauma. Most people who are naturally aligned with their Healer energy really dislike seeing disharmony, pain, or suffering. They are often dissatisfied with the way the world is and how human beings treat each other.

Society often doesn't value the Healer in each of us very highly, perhaps because so many people are unconscious of their own pain. To recognize the importance of healing would be to admit that there's something deep within us as a species that is broken.

The exception to this is physical pain. Perhaps that is why medical doctors are considered by society to be the highest form of Healer and are usually well compensated for their work. Others like nurses, therapists, coaches, social workers, and energy practitioners tend to get paid lower wages and are often not recognized for the incredible contribution they bring to the world. And, of course, a lot of healing is done by people who don't get paid at all, like parents and friends. Police officers, firefighters, schoolteachers, and just plain old good neighbors also do their fair share of healing work. In fact, many of the professionals go into these vocations because they want to make things better for people and serve their communities.

We all have Healer energy inside us, but not everyone knows how to recognize it or what to do with it. My own Healer energy has always been strong, but I didn't always understand what to do with it in order to help others.

Once, when I was in middle school, some other students were being disrespectful to a teacher. I could feel a knot form in my stomach and my heart hurt. I thought: *Can't you see you're hurting her feelings?* That part of me—the instinctive part of me that wanted everyone to feel okay—was my Healer energy. At the time, however, I didn't know what to do with that feeling or how to manage it, although seeing other people in obvious discomfort or pain (whether physical or emotional) traumatized me. Later in life, as I developed professionally in areas that utilize this energy, I had to do a lot of work with my own Healer energy to recognize that this sensitivity is actually a healthy part of my calling. Being sensitive to others isn't a weakness—just an unrealized potential.

When people don't manage their Healer energy in a balanced way, they may find themselves feeling an excess of negative emotions, because those who are more naturally in tune with Healer energy are especially sensitive to other people's pain. They are commonly referred to as empaths, because they intuitively absorb what others are feeling. Unfortunately, it is not uncommon to see those with sensitive Healer energy lose the ability to live happy and balanced lives due to their sensitivity. Other people's pain can be overwhelming. Because there is an almost infinite amount of pain in the world, there never seems to be an end to the cycle of absorbing and releasing it for these sensitives. And that can be exhausting if not properly balanced.

The hardest lesson for the Healer to learn is thus to establish and maintain healthy boundaries. They must learn to face pain in a neutral and compassionate way and to let go of self-judgment around being sensitive to Healer energy. Making sure that this part of them is balanced and healthy is essential when it comes to awakening to their highest potential.

## The Healer in Balance

Healers who are truly grounded in their authenticity understand at a deep level that people can't be forced or coerced into healing. This would be a subtle form of manipulation or aggression. Healing has to arise naturally through personal growth.

Here are some of the characteristics of balanced Healer energy:

- Sensitivity

- Empathy

- The ability to listen

- Compassion

- Ethical living

- Understanding

- Affinity to nature

- Emotional intelligence

- Sexual sensitivity

- A desire to fix what is broken

- A need for wholeness

- A desire to heal the planet

For materialists, some healing modalities and the personalities who come with them can seem "woo-woo," irrational, or overly emotional. And sometimes this is for good reason. When I started my healing training in Hawaii, my nickname was Cosmic, because I was so ungrounded and always had my head in the stars. I didn't enjoy having a job or operating within the normal constructs of society. And that attitude bothered my more mainstream friends.

Part of the dynamic for me was that I just didn't enjoy the material and physical world that much and yearned to live on a more spiritual plane. But another important factor for me was that, every time I felt someone else's pain, I just wanted to float up off the planet to avoid it. My teachers had to constantly and gently remind me to ground myself and stay present, even in the midst of pain.

Later, as I began teaching spiritual healers, I noticed that many of them came through the door just as I had—ungrounded, idealistic, and holding on to other people's pain. To be a healthy Healer, however, it's important to remember that you also live in the physical world. One realm is not "higher" or "better" than another. Healers who feel disdain for materialistic people or for the material world end up falling into the same negative energy as those they look down on.

Healers can learn to embrace both ends of this spectrum, however, and to validate every experience and worldview. This is how they become truly successful. It's okay to have your head in the clouds as long as your feet are firmly planted on the ground.

## The Healer in Deficit

I've known many Healers who avoid awakening their true healing energy. It's not uncommon for someone who is sensitive to take the attitude that there is too much pain in themselves or in the world to deal with, so it's just not worth the effort. Their lack of self-worth may reflect a belief that either they aren't capable of healing themselves or others, or that no one is worth healing.

Those who avoid their own healing abilities can easily fall into depression and lose hope that things in their own lives or in the world can ever change. They may believe that things are too broken to be reconciled. This pessimism, in some ways, stems from deep-seated pain. On the deepest level, the Healer in deficit believes that pain or conflict can't be healed, because they themselves can't be healed or loved.

Deficient Healer energy can manifest as:

• Selfishness

• Pessimistic view of human nature

- Fear of experiencing pain

- Apathy

- Feelings of isolation

- Cold energy

- Feelings of being victimized

- Inability to process emotion in a healthy way

- Trouble tapping into empathy

- Inability to heal trauma

- Difficulty listening to the concerns of others

This isn't an exhaustive list, but it should give you a sense of what a deficient Healer may be experiencing.

There are three main causes for a deficit in Healer energy. All are rooted in fear—fear of pain, fear of involvement, and fear of sexuality.

### *Fear of Pain*

From time to time, we all harden our hearts in order to protect ourselves from pain. Healers who do this risk creating an external shell around themselves to protect their feelings and, in the process, lose touch with the deeper parts of their being. From the outside, these people may not look like Healers at all. I've seen many strong, externally tough people take this energetic posture. They create an aura of strength that says: "I don't need anyone's help," or "Emotions are for wimps," or "I'm perfectly fine and I'm not in need of any healing at all." They may even be offended by offers of help or resistant when asked to help others. If part of a soul's destiny is to heal, however, and that soul avoids the calling, misery will likely follow.

There's an old adage that says: "Healer, heal thyself." When you truly heal yourself, you conquer the fear of pain. When you open to helping others, you heal the deficient Healer in you and bring meaning to your life.

### Fear of Involvement

Sometimes Healers in deficit may deny their vocational calling in order to hide from their destiny. They may take a safe job, or one that isolates them from dealing with other people's problems, so that they don't have to experience the anxiety or pain that many human beings carry with them day-to-day. The world is full of people who have avoided their calling because they were afraid of something. For the Healer in deficit, it's often a fear of pain. But avoiding pain is just another form of pain. By avoiding their calling, they are creating the pain of missing their purpose.

As you awaken your inner Healer, you will find parts of you that have been neglected, stuck, or broken. Handle each part with care and get the professional help you need to heal. As you find wholeness inside yourself on every level, your presence will become a healing for all of humanity, and happiness will naturally flower from your heart—from the inside out.

### Fear of Sexuality

Sexuality tends to be simultaneously suppressed and abused in Western society. Sexual trauma, body image issues, and the accompanying feelings of shame and guilt have all combined to create one of the most misunderstood and painful energies with which we have to deal.

Shame, guilt, repression, and other forms of blocked energy can lock power and pleasure down in the lower body, warp the sense of self, and stop life energy from flowing through the rest of the system. This can also block the Healer's potential healing power. My experience in counseling has shown me that one place where many Healers tend to hold on to an enormous amount of pain is in their sexual space.

When I was in my early twenties, I had read many books on Tantra and sexuality, but the information was all stuck in my head. Then one day, in the mountains in Thailand, I had a synchronistic encounter with a wonderful Tantra teacher and decided to participate in one of her retreats. From her, I learned how to look inward to see where my own shame and guilt lay and where poor communication with my partner led to blocked energy. Most of all, she showed me how much collective pain humanity holds around sexual energy.

Many Healers find, as they truly heal, that this part of themselves starts to flower in a new way. Practices like Tantra, Kama Sutra, Kundalini, Orgasmic Meditation, and other forms of more evolved sexuality will be necessary for the healing and evolution of human beings. Healers have an important role to play in this area, but they must first unlock their own potential.

## The Healer in Excess

When Healers move toward excess, they may express characteristics like excessive worrying, trying to heal everyone else but not themselves, being anxious about safety, or not establishing healthy boundaries with negative people. They may feel a need to sacrifice themselves, to become martyrs, to give excessively, and to deplete their own energy by always putting others first. These are all telltale signs that their Healer energy is out of balance and in excess.

Other ways in which excessive Healer energy manifests include:

- A constant need to fix others

- A tendency to be out of the body

- Uncontrollable anxiety or worry

- A tendency to absorb others' pain

- Discomfort in awkward or aggressive situations

- Avoidance of confrontation

- A belief they can fix everything

- Depending too much on validation from helping others

- Poor establishment and maintenance of boundaries

- Attracting people in pain

- Always getting drawn into drama

- Uncontrollable outward flow of energy

On a practical level, an excess of Healer energy is often rooted in four main behaviors: enabling dysfunction, neglecting boundaries, falling prey to what I call the "savior syndrome," and going over to the "dark side."

### Enabling Dysfunction

Some Healers in excess may find themselves enabling dysfunctional or self-destructive friends or family instead of helping them see the consequences of their behavior—by providing financial support, for example.

When I was living in Hawaii, I badly needed a place to live and I just couldn't seem to find something to rent. A friend of mine was also looking for housing at the same time. I had already helped him find a job. When I finally did find something, I succumbed to an excess of Healer energy and let him have the house because I didn't want to see him suffer. The problem was, I didn't take into account the underlying issues he had at the time. And, of course, I also neglected my own needs.

Eventually the situation deteriorated and my friend became increasingly unstable and angry, and we weren't able to continue our friendship—which led to me taking over the lease to the house and moving in. When this happened, I finally realized that I had, in fact, created this entire set of circumstances because I had been trying to heal my friend's life when he wasn't in a place to receive the healing.

### Neglecting Boundaries

When Healers are in excess, they lose touch with rational decision-making and are easily pulled into other people's problems and drama, attempting to deliver healing at all costs. They may let others pour their pain out onto them without maintaining safe boundaries. Or they may give up an important opportunity so someone else can have it instead. Interestingly, the friend I described above was also a practicing spiritual healer. I believe he had absorbed so much pain from other people that it had created an imbalance in his own energies. When my own anger around the situation subsided, I recognized that I needed to establish boundaries with him. I needed to feel compassion for him, but I didn't need to *fix* him.

Because Healers in excess are great at giving but have a hard time receiving, they often find themselves unconsciously looking for validation in the wrong places. So, as strange as this sounds, they need to learn how to *heal their Healer* by working through old trauma or pain and cultivating a deeper sense of self-worth. A Healer who is awakening out of excess needs to realize that, when expressed from a place of balance, giving *is* receiving. There is no loss of energy in this kind of true exchange. A soul can never truly be fulfilled until it learns how to give in a healthy way within appropriate boundaries.

### The Savior Syndrome

Another sign that you are suffering from an excess of Healer energy is a belief that you are the "savior" who can resolve or heal someone else's issues. Others may have answers that have healing value, of course. But Healers in excess cannot admit this. They may see themselves as a savior, or even a martyr, engaged in an epic struggle to heal everyone they meet. At first, this kind of excessive healing energy may seem as if it puts other people first. But when you look more closely, you see that it's really all about the Healer's own ego. When your identity and self-validation lie in the value you bring by healing others, everything becomes personal.

I'm familiar with this type of excess because I definitely experienced it in myself. When I started doing professional spiritual counseling and healings, I thought that I could fix everyone. I set out to prove my value to the world by fixing every broken person I came across. But soon, the external validation that I needed began to overshadow the actual needs of my clients.

I had to take a step back and recognize that I wasn't the best fit for everyone. Nor was I the best spiritual healer in the world. I had to begin to find my validation on the inside, instead of from healing other people's pain. If this sounds familiar to you, it may be time to check in with your own healing patterns and ask why you have fallen into them. We often overheal either because, on a deep level, we're trying to hide our own pain or we believe that, if we help others, they will give us the acceptance and love we seek.

### The Dark Side

Healers who turn toward the darkness may have experienced excessive amounts of pain they couldn't handle, wounds they couldn't heal, or sensitivities they couldn't manage.

These broken Healers can find their depression, anger, apathy, or pain so unbearable that they may even turn on themselves. Instead of healing, their pain takes over as their primary identity, and this may lead them to try feeding on more pain, looking everywhere for more of it to absorb.

To be clear, we all have a dark side. And sometimes the more we try to cultivate the "good" side of ourselves, the more we end up merely covering up the darkness. But truly good-hearted Healers don't have to be "good." When they heal, goodness arises naturally out of their being as a by-product and expression of their soul.

## Back to Balance

In order to be happy and fulfilled, we must learn to use our Healer energy to *heal ourselves first*. We have a natural tendency to focus our attention outward, because it is usually easier to deal with other people's pain rather than our own. But Healers must turn the healing toward themselves first, and with self-compassion. Only after they heal themselves can they radiate healing energy outward in a healthy way.

It's also important for Healers to come to terms with the way the world is in the present moment. There are so many problems in the world that can trigger us—war, disease, violence, tragedy, injustice—and it is critical for Healers to understand that they can't help the world if they exist in a state of debilitating rage, despair, numbness, or surrender.

### Meditation to Balance Healing Energy

We can talk about healing until the cows come home, but the real work here is done on the *inside* of your being. This is where the true healing takes place. This meditation may help to take you to a place of inner balance.

> **Step 1:** As you gently close your eyes and relax into your body, begin by asking a very simple question: "What is one area in me that needs healing in order for my inner Healer to rise to its potential?"

**Step 2:** Notice that, even though you can have thousands of memories and ideas related to one topic, when you ask the right question, breathe slowly, and sit still, just one important thought-energy rises to the surface, like an air bubble coming to the top of a body of water.

**Step 3:** Reach down with your hand and scoop up that bubble, which contains an energy and image that pertain to what your being is truly calling to be healed. As you notice the theme, whether it's related to relationships, self-worth, trauma, sensitivity, or anything else you are working on healing, you also recognize that this energy will help you awaken your Healer. And it will also, at some point, help you to heal others.

**Step 4:** See if you can embrace how you feel with the same attitude you would have toward someone you love deeply who is in pain—with compassion and care. You don't have to fix anything or figure anything out; just see if you can feel a sense of acceptance toward whatever you're finding difficult to embrace. And if you can't welcome this part of yourself, see if you can accept the part of you that can't accept it.

**Step 5:** Envision a beautiful golden light entering through the top of your head and shining down on every part of you. Notice that the light makes no judgment; it shines and warms everything equally. Only the mind breaks things into parts and stories.

**Step 6:** As you fill with this golden light and your energy begins to shift, you get a subtle sense of the direction in which your inner Healer wants to move. Who around you could benefit from your healing, from your light? Extend that light out to them, and see them coming into wholeness and out of judgment or invalidation.

**Step 7:** Notice that other people's healing is also your healing, and your healing is theirs. You are truly beginning to rise to your healing potential, and it didn't take changing who you are. All you had to do was embrace and accept how you feel, and not see those feelings as a problem. When you're ready, slowly open your eyes.

Spend some time with your journal. Is there a specific memory or image that comes to you of a time when you were in balance, freely giving and receiving? Is there a place in your body that feels less stressed? What does that feel like?

### Healer Self-Reflection

As always, meditation is most effective when followed by self-reflection. Ask yourself these questions to help you assess your deficient Healer tendencies:

- Do you avoid deep relationships so you don't have to feel other people's pain?

- Do you find yourself hiding out at home to avoid the heavy energies of the world?

- Do you find yourself putting up unhealthy emotional walls or excessive boundaries with people in your life to avoid their energy?

- Do you think that trying to help people or change the world is a losing battle? Do you think you should even try?

- Do you sometimes feel disconnected or lacking in empathy for people who are struggling or in pain?

Now ask yourself these questions to help identify your excessive Healer tendencies:

- Do you notice that you tend to absorb other people's pain uncontrollably?

- Do you have a hard time telling the difference between your feelings and other people's feelings?

- Do you tend to not maintain good boundaries when it comes to other people asking you for help when it's inappropriate?

- Do you find too much of your personal value in healing others?

- Do you have an easier time giving energy than receiving it?

Finally, try answering these questions as you work to cultivate balanced Healer energy:

- What inside of me needs healing in order to grow?

- How much of other people's pain have I been unconsciously trying to manage or heal?

- What pain inside of me is attracting the pain of others?

- What dynamics or beliefs keep me from establishing and maintaining healthy boundaries?

- How would I behave differently if I were a healthy Healer?

- As my Healer energy rises to its potential, how do I want to share it with the world?

### Healer Goals

Consider the difference between how Healer energy works internally and externally. Then see if you can come up with three ways in which you can apply your Healer energy to your life on an internal level. For example:

- Let go of some old anger.

- Heal my inner child.

- Heal from an old relationship.

Now write down three ways in which you can apply your Healer energy to your life on an external level. For example:

- Be a better listener.

- Practice more hands-on healing.

- Be a healthy space-holder for others.

### *Healer Action: Authentic Listening*

Giving someone your undivided, compassionate attention can be an enormous gift, not only to that person, but also to your inner Healer. Authentic listening requires more than being utterly present to another person in the moment. It also requires that you be aware of your own inner monologue, neither absorbing and coopting their emotions or projecting your own emotions onto them. Practicing this skill is a great way to balance your Healer energy.

This exercise is hard to schedule, but try to be on the lookout for opportunities to listen actively when others tell you their story—for instance, when your partner or roommate talks about events at work, or when a long-distance friend gives you an update on how things are going. You can also seek out circumstances in which you can naturally engage in conversations with relative strangers during the course of your day if you feel moved to do so, although introverts may not be as enthusiastic about this as extroverts may be. Try chatting with the person seated next to you on a plane or in a long line at the grocery store. Granted that most of these conversations may not delve too deeply into people's emotional lives, but you can still practice active listening even when others are sharing mundane details about their professions or hobbies.

Here are few key practices that can help you implement active listening:

- Remain in the present moment yourself—i.e., not thinking of other errands you need to run or tasks you need to accomplish.

- Make eye contact with the other person and signal through your body language (nodding, smiling, etc.) that you are engaged.

- Share common experiences or even advice, although this can sometimes signal a preoccupation with your own experiences or expertise (a sign of Healer excess). Sometimes it's better to signal your presence and interest without telling your own stories.

If you are involved in a more emotional conversation, paraphrasing can often help others feel that they are being authentically heard, while simultaneously allowing you to engage more fully with them by confirming that you understand what is being said. We all have our own preconceived ideas about the world, and we often think we know what we are hearing when, in fact, we may only have a partial (or even entirely incorrect) understanding of the situation.

Here are a few examples of paraphrasing:

- *Your friend*: I had an awful day. I had so much to do and I ran around all day trying to get everything on my to-do list done. And I feel as if I still didn't really accomplish anything. I never get a break.

- *You*: It sounds as if you are really stressed-out and exhausted.

- *Your friend*: Yes, exactly! I am so stressed-out. I probably need to take a day off and relax.

Paraphrasing also helps you maintain emotional boundaries. By naming the emotional reality you see in someone else, you become more aware of whether you are absorbing those emotions yourself. This can help you uncover areas in which you may want to work to shore up your personal boundaries.

You may want to record any experiences or feelings that come up for you while working with active listening in your journal. Healer energy is a deeply emotional energy, and there is a lot to work with here for many.

# Chapter 5

# The Warrior

*A warrior does not give up what he loves,*
*he finds the love in what he does.*

—Dan Millman

Warrior energy embodies discipline, focus, and commitment. When at its peak potential, Warrior energy becomes the part of you that is willing to exert consistent healthy effort, overcome fear of death, go directly at the truth, and cut through the jungle of illusion with its sword of discretion.

Warriors are loyal to their mission, courageous in the face of challenges, and able to see through the seduction of distractions. Alert, humble, and honest, Warriors train and perfect their efforts and discipline with integrity so they can handle whatever life puts in front of them.

When I first started practicing meditation, I wasn't particularly good at it. By which I mean that, when I closed my eyes, I wasn't suddenly awash in a waterfall of bliss or enlightened thoughts. I struggled with meditation, as many do. But I was relentless when it came to the *practice*. I sat over and over again. I sat when I was tired. I sat when I was frustrated. I sat when I was angry and depressed. I sat when I was afraid. Somehow, the Warrior energy in me decided that sitting still was my battle, my journey. In that persistence, I eventually found inner stillness. And from that stillness, I eventually experienced tremendous breakthroughs. My thoughts gave up and fell away; my resistance disappeared; I found peace.

Of course, I'm not perfect in my meditation practice. It is something I still struggle with. But the discipline and determination of sitting despite struggle and imperfection are emblematic of the Warrior energy that we all need to access in these moments to remind ourselves that nothing is achieved without great focus. The Warrior defeats resistance at its own game by admitting the issue and facing it with resilience.

## The Warrior in Balance

In modern culture, Warrior energy supports the lives of soldiers, athletes, monks, and fitness instructors. Society tends to hold soldiers and athletes in particularly high esteem. When LeBron James shoots a game-winning shot, or a Navy Seal team captures a bad guy under impossible conditions, those accomplishments—the perfection of the Warrior's craft—are cheered by others. We all value the mastery of a skill, which is where the Warrior energy excels.

Sometimes achieving our full Warrior potential just means showing up consistently, every day, in the face of adversity. At other times, it means breaking through limitations and barriers that seem impossible to conquer. Breathwork teacher Wim Hof, also known as the Iceman, is a great example of the Warrior energy taking form. When he was a young man, his wife committed suicide and left him to raise his four children alone. After working through deep grief and searching his soul for answers, one day he decided to jump into a freezing river in the Netherlands and began building resistance to the cold through breathwork and meditation.

Utilizing these techniques, Hof eventually broke numerous world records and performed a number of astonishing feats, including climbing past Mount Everest's "Death Zone" dressed in shorts. While not all of us need to demonstrate our Warrior energy through the achievement of such amazing feats, Hof's accomplishments are outward manifestations of his commitment to push past limitation and pain. That is how his soul expresses its Warrior energy.

When Warrior energy reaches its peak, individuals often achieve what modern psychologists call a "flow state"—some call it "being in the zone." This state of awareness, this centered presence, arises out of a combination of mastery and focus. Like musicians who, after practicing for years with extraordinary effort, begin to play at an advanced level without any seeming effort at all, Warriors operate in flow. They make confident choices; they finish projects under enormous pressure; they score a game-winning goal. Or perhaps they just sit still in meditation through pain and resistance when the body wants to give up.

Those with balanced Warrior energy are:

- Decisive

- Direct

- Structured

- Truthful

- Confident

- Humble

- Alert

- Disciplined

- Consistent

- Honorable

- Loyal

- Protective

- Grounded

- Courageous

- Certain

You may think that you don't have Warrior energy, that you are a soft, sensitive meditator. But Warrior energy, just like the other six energies, exists in each of us in unique ways.

Your Warrior energy may reach its potential by cutting through the chaos in your own head, or by managing the illusions and problems other people throw at you at work. It may come through as you hold on to your integrity in precarious situations that could cause you to lose something of value. Or it may manifest as a deeply disciplined regimen that helps you stay grounded through a cancer diagnosis and subsequent treatment.

Balanced Warriors understand that, in the material world in which we live, effort, discipline, and commitment are vital to maintaining a stable foundation of energy. The Buddha, it is said, exerted great effort, failing again and again. He ate a grain of rice a day;

he lay on a bed of nails; he lived outside with nothing to shelter him; he meditated for endless hours searching for enlightenment. And all that effort—all those failures—finally led him to find what he later described as the middle path. His Warrior energy gave him the will to sit still under the Bodhi tree and face his demons.

After the Buddha attained his awakened state and began teaching, he asked his followers to commit to great discipline. They wore robes; they shaved their heads; they ate little food. They walked from village to village, begging. They meditated for many hours and kept to strict rules regarding sexuality. All of these commitments took energy and effort. But how is it that a man who found enlightenment by letting go, by surrendering to the truth in the moment, by shedding all the conventions of society, went on to ask his students to commit to rigid discipline? He simply understood the stages and energies of growth necessary to develop as a human being. He didn't ask his students to begin where he ended; he asked them to begin where he had started.

## The Warrior in Deficit

Those with deficient Warrior energy may be indecisive, afraid, apathetic, unfocused, or display a lack of integrity. Today, people expend their efforts in so many places at once, and spend so much time online, that their energy ends up being scattered. It has no focus or direction. It has no clear intent.

I think our society has, for the most part, lost its sense of what real Warrior energy can be. We watch movies where *other* people are heroes; we go to sporting events and wear jerseys with *other* people's names on our backs. We have become spectators rather than players. It is, after all, safer to be a spectator—to watch and criticize from a distance. But there is no *life* in that. Warriors choose to become the heroes of their own stories, not spectators of someone else's.

When Warrior energy is in deficit, we become:

• Indecisive

• Afraid

• Unethical

• Stubborn

• Apathetic

• Unfocused

• Scattered

• Dishonest

• Anxious

- Weak

- Disloyal

- Dishonorable

Three patterns that can suppress Warrior energy and keep it out of balance are lack of discipline, lack of self-esteem, and lack of structure.

### Lack of Discipline

So many people lack purpose in today's society. They go to work to make a living so they can pay the rent, buy food, and pay for entertainment. Then they repeat the cycle over and over again, slowly dying a little bit more each day. They wish they had the time or money to do this or that, but it's not the money or the time that stops them. It's a lack of discipline, an inability to follow through, a fear of failure, or a lack of belief in themselves.

### Lack of Self-Esteem

Those with deficient Warrior energy often suffer from "victim consciousness" and a paralyzing lack of self-esteem. They often feel that the circumstances of their lives aren't fair. But true Warriors know that life is fair in its own hidden way, because everyone's purpose is different. They know that comparing their path to another's path is the wrong way to look at things.

### Lack of Structure

Sometimes people use the need for spontaneity and flow as an excuse to avoid discipline and structure. Many artists and spiritual seekers avoid feeding their inner Warrior because it seems antithetical to the flow and movement of creativity. But Warrior energy is often exactly what is missing in their quest for success. Sometimes the greatest creative or entrepreneurial minds just need a bit more structure to give their creations form. When Warrior energy is in deficit, they come up against the energy of fear or avoidance instead.

When I started my online training program, I had no structure to my business. I recorded meditations, dealt with the parts of the business that I enjoyed, and avoided dealing with the parts I didn't understand. My progress was slow. Eventually, I hired a business coach to help me see what was missing and to bring structure to the process.

My business might never have gotten off the ground without that coach helping me to see my weak points—particularly the technology wall I kept banging my head against. My coach made me realize how inefficient and undisciplined I was. I was approaching my business with the mind of an Artist and a Creator, but I was missing the Warrior energy needed to see the project through. It took another Warrior to teach and inspire me.

To heal deficient Warrior energy, we sometimes need real honest reflection, outside inspiration, and a recognition of where and what we fear. Don't allow indecision and indecisiveness to stop you from growing. Use those energies to inform you about where you lack focus and call on your inner Warrior to get you to the other side.

## The Warrior in Excess

To truly embrace Warrior energy, you must understand focus, effort, and action. But Warriors in excess can become obsessed with that focus and forget about what's truly important. They can neglect their love for the game, the craft, or the journey and turn toward a love of outcomes instead. Warriors in excess can become obsessive about winning, defending, conquering, and being better than everyone else. They may feel a constant need to prove some kind of superior skill or strength. They may form an identity around being "the best" and view anyone who challenges them as an enemy.

Warriors in excess may also become lost in excessive effort, believing that every problem is a nail that needs a hammer. Or that the effort used to solve one issue can be used to solve all issues. These excessive efforts, which may at first help launch them out of the gravitational pull of laziness or apathy, can later become self-destructive forces in the growth process.

Warriors in excess risk becoming:

- Overly competitive

- Controlling

- Workaholics

- Aggressive

- Ego-driven

- Obsessed with winning

- Prone to exert too much effort

- Narcissistic

- Lacking in compassion

- Excessively goal-driven

There are three behaviors that can keep your Warrior energy in excess and lead to a lack of balance: what I call "110-percentism," narcissism, and lack of spontaneity.

### "110-Percentism"

Warriors in excess may start identifying as people who always work hard—who always give 110 percent. This can lead to the belief that, if something isn't hard, it isn't worth doing. But this conviction can become a subtle form of avoidance, or even violence toward themselves. It's easy to use effort as an excuse to override emotions that need to be felt, conversations that need to be had, and failures that need to be accepted.

### Narcissism

Narcissism can also lead to a Warrior energy that is out of control. Excess Warrior energy can manifest as an inability to be a team player, as a thirst for power, or as bullying. Warriors in excess tend to judge people who don't exhibit their Warrior energy in the same way they do—perhaps by focusing on saving the trees through benign means. These judgments can turn them toward verbal or even physical violence, anger, or hate. When Warriors fuel their egos by controlling others, they can easily descend to a lower level of consciousness.

### Lack of Spontaneity

Excess Warrior energy can also take the form of a continual need to give everything in life structure and discipline, even where spontaneity and ease are called for. This can cause the Warrior in excess to become stiff, ideological, and devoid of compassion.

When Warriors forget why they got into their field or interest in the first place and lose themselves in ambition, it may be a clear sign that their Warrior energy is out of balance. As a Warrior, you must never lose sight of your own meaning and purpose. Remember: Warrior energy, like all energies, exists to be of service to the soul and to humanity.

## Back to Balance

It's very likely that there are areas where you have little trouble accessing your Warrior energy and others where you may continually struggle to do so. Or you may experience situations in which you tend to overdo your Warrior energy and cause suffering in the process. It's important to remember that being honest with where you actually *are* is the first step to bringing yourself into balance. If you have apathetic tendencies, be honest with yourself about them. If you often try to overcome invalidation or fear through excess effort or by attempting to override your feelings, be honest with those energies as well. Radical self-honesty will help set you free.

When I was fifteen, just about a year before my first deep realization with meditation, my parents sent me off to a Russian ice hockey camp that required that you speak Russian. My parents were immigrants from Belarus, so I grew up speaking Russian, but I was probably the worst Russian speaker at the camp. I quickly became close friends with a player there who didn't speak a word of English, yet somehow we hit it off.

That player ended up being the first pick in the NHL draft when he was just eighteen. He won a gold medal for Russia at the Olympics and became one of the best hockey players in the world. He was probably the first person in my life who stood as a clear example of someone living up to their full Warrior potential.

Playing next to him, I quickly realized that being a professional hockey player wasn't in the cards for me. But I also learned how to focus and master a skill by applying the right amount of effort. I used that experience, and still do to this day, when I'm building a course, growing a business, or working on some other creative endeavor. His example motivates me toward my goals.

### Meditation to Balance Warrior Energy

Warrior energy needs focus and direction. It's the part of your nature that helps you accomplish goals.

This meditation can help you set goals for manifesting a balanced Warrior energy in your life.

**Step 1:** As you step into meditation with your eyes closed, see if you can straighten your spine and really focus on sitting still. Notice that true Warrior energy is not tense, but focused and relaxed.

**Step 2:** Imagine yourself sitting in front of a calm lake, looking down at the water. As you peer into the lake, you notice a bubble from down below slowly begin to rise to the surface. You put your hand in the water and scoop it up. With an open palm, you look inside it. There, you find a clear image of what you look like when you are tapping into your balanced inner Warrior.

**Step 3:** See if you can notice how the deep essence of your Warrior is not just a means to an end, like being more focused or assertive, but rather a true reflection of the part of your soul that isn't afraid to show up in the world and put in the effort to accomplish your deepest goals as a human being.

**Step 4:** Ask yourself if you're truly ready to shed any fear of failure, any inflated or deflated sense of self, and be a true, humble Warrior. This is not an option, but a calling from deep within your being.

**Step 5:** Begin to notice that your Warrior energy has a certain tone and even color to it. You can sense that color around your body. And you recognize that you can call on this aspect of yourself anytime you need to.

**Step 6:** Consider what life goal your inner Warrior wants to focus on. How can you apply this energy to achieve this goal?

**Step 7:** See yourself achieving this goal with the right amount of effort and with total focus. Feel it in your body. As you integrate your inner Warrior into the rest of your being, know that there is nothing you can't achieve.

### Warrior Self-Reflection

You can only balance your inner Warrior by looking within. Ask yourself these questions to determine if your Warrior energy is in deficit:

- Do you have a hard time focusing your energy on important tasks or achieving goals?

- Do you often let yourself slip into apathy or laziness when it comes to finishing projects?

- Do you tend to give in to fear when it comes to taking a risk to get something you want?

- Do you avoid taking care of your nutrition? Do you not get enough physical exercise or enough consistent sleep?

- Do you wish you were more consistent and relentless in your pursuit of living your best life?

Now ask yourself these questions to determine if your Warrior energy is in excess:

- Do you find yourself overworking in order to override your feelings or prove yourself to the world?

- Do you have an inherent belief that more effort is always the solution?

- Do you have an insatiable need to win, always be right, or conquer?

- Do you need to experience extreme danger or competition to feel alive?

Finally, consider these questions as you commit to cultivating a balanced Warrior energy:

- In what way have I been avoiding my inner power?

- Do I take good care of my physical body with exercise and nutrition?

- When a moment calls for decision and action, do I normally take it swiftly or spend excessive time weighing different factors?

- Do I often find myself struggling against life with too much effort? If so, how?

- If I were living up to my Warrior potential, how would I show up differently in the world?

### Warrior Goals

Consider the difference between how Warrior energy works internally and externally. Then see if you can come up with three ways in which you can apply your Warrior energy to your life on an internal level. For example:

- Harness more self-confidence.

- Stop hiding my power.

- Exert less effort.

Now write down three ways in which you can apply your Warrior energy to your life on an external level. For example:

- Engage in consistent physical exercise.

- Be more proactive at work and take action.

- Fight for a special cause.

### Warrior Action: Commit—Then Show Up

Warriors make firm decisions and then show up for them. To exercise your Warrior energy, think of an area in your life that you have wanted to improve for some time, but have been struggling with due to a lack of discipline—for instance, a regular exercise program, a regular spiritual or meditation practice, or regular local volunteer work. Once you have identified the area in which you want to work, choose one clear action you can take within that area and set a realistic goal.

For example, let's say you want to establish a regular program of physical exercise. This is something that many people struggle with. There are, of course, many different kinds of physical exercise and most health professionals will tell you that the best one for you will depend on a number of factors. For our example here, let's set the goal of walking or running for twenty minutes every day for two weeks at the same time each morning.

Now comes the most difficult part of the exercise, of course—you have to show up! This is where you need to dig deep and summon up your Warrior energy. Make a firm and unimpeachable decision to wake up every morning at the same time for two weeks, put on your walking clothes and shoes, and go for a walk or run for twenty minutes. Tell yourself that the decision is final. Commit to showing up every day for this. Write your goal down somewhere if that helps you. It is important; it is in line with your personal goals; you have decided to do it. And you will.

Once you are on your walk, relish the feeling of your Warrior energy surging through you—the energy that helped you get to this place. You may even begin to notice that you get into the "flow state" as you walk. This is a sure sign that the Warrior in you is balanced and thriving.

# Chapter 6

# The Lover

*For small creatures such as we, the*
*vastness is bearable only through love.*
—Carl Sagan

One of the deepest forms of spiritual growth is the realization that the fabric of reality is woven with the energy of love. Every great sage across time and tradition has gently pointed us toward this truth—that love and connection lie behind the doorway of the heart. We feel this on a personal level when we love our families, our partners, or our friends. We feel it on a cosmic scale when we experience a oneness with all humanity, with nature, with the planet, or with the universe.

People who embody their Lover energy tend to have big sensitive hearts and to create space in their lives for others from all walks of life. They are motivated by the energy of acceptance and connection, of caring and compassion, and by consideration for others. These are all hallmarks of the Lover.

The dark side of this sensitivity and compassion can manifest as loneliness, isolation, rejection, heartbreak, or loss. These experiences can seem like a curse to the Lover, because there is nothing more painful than the loss or rejection of love. But when we understand Lover energy from a deeper perspective, however, we can learn to turn a hardened rock of pain into a diamond of love. Often, those who have been through the most hardship and come out the other side are the most compassionate and understanding people in the world.

## The Lover in Balance

On a spiritual level, the opening of the heart and the awakening of balanced Lover energy transcends personal relationships. Love becomes impersonal. Love becomes an expression of oneness.

Once when I was attending a retreat, I found myself bound up by tension and confusion while I was deep in meditation. The teacher had asked us not to move even an inch as we meditated, and I was struggling with that. Then suddenly, since I couldn't fidget my way out of my feelings, I just let go. I surrendered to the situation and accepted how I felt without trying to change it. A deep inner peace opened up in my heart, and I could feel all of life pulsating through me.

After the meditation, I got up and walked outside. I could feel the ground, the trees, the sky, and the stars. This connection was impersonal, and yet *very* personal. At that moment, the words of all the sages of the past made sense to me. Their descriptions of oneness and love as the nature of reality became real to me, not just concepts in my spiritual library.

There is an inherent ability in the Lover energy to open to this kind of awareness, but it is often covered up by pain. And so the job of the Lover is to heal the heart with the balm of acceptance and to open to life.

Those with balanced Lover energy tend to value relationships and to work to resolve conflicts. They are:

- Authentic

- Compassionate

- Caring

- Openhearted

- Accepting

- Sensitive

- Honest

- Purpose-driven

- Nurturing

- Loyal

- Kind

Our life lessons to balance Lover energy aren't always easy, however. We all experience the deep sadness of loss. The certainty of loss, which lies at the core of the Buddha's four noble truths, is something we all have to face at some point in our lives. And grief can break open even the most hardened of hearts.

Unfortunately many people wait until the moment of a loved one's death, or even their own death, to acknowledge their feelings, to forgive, and to appreciate life. But when grief goes unacknowledged, it can become the Lover's Achilles' heel. It can sink a heart to the bottom of the ocean of despair and drown the Lover in pain. Processing grief in a positive way—with a therapist, in meditation, or through some other spiritual or psychological practice—is thus vital to having healthy and balanced Lover energy.

To awaken to life, you must dare to live. To live, you must love. And to love, you must own and heal your heart. There are countless stories of people who have had near-death experiences and come out the other side with a different set of priorities. Their newfound second chance awakens them to what's truly important, and they start to live.

Love and passion that are born of the heart shine a light onto our life's path. They help us find who we truly are and what we should be doing in the world. We find our purpose in the heart center. That is to say, we find our purpose, and our most meaningful understandings, when we balance our Lover energy.

## The Lover in Deficit

Those experiencing a deficiency in Lover energy may find themselves feeling that their hearts are closed. They may avoid relationships, deny deep feelings, or neglect real communication or commitment. They may decide, consciously or unconsciously, that, since anything they love will eventually be lost, it is better to stay safe and not get hurt. In fact, they may decide that it's better to avoid loving connections altogether.

Deficient Lover energy can manifest as a tendency to stay single or to be trapped in shallow, superficial relationships. Or it may be reflected in children who continue to take from their parents after they are grown, giving nothing in return or in those who use other people to get ahead. Lovers in deficit may believe that the world is made up of cold, violent beings who only mean them harm. They often feel that it's better to remain isolated, alone, and safe.

A deficiency in Lover energy also manifests as:

- A closed heart

- Selfishness

- Judgmental attitudes

- Difficulty giving or receiving love

- Difficulty communicating feelings

- Disconnection from emotions

- Disillusionment

- Lack of self-worth

- Lack of self-love

- Feelings of invalidation

- Difficulty finding purpose

- Perceptions that the world is cold and uncaring

- Difficulty trusting

- Manipulativeness

- A tendency to use others

There are three main emotional states that can contribute to a deficiency in Lover energy: regret, fear of rejection, and lack of validation.

### Regret

Regret is a deep wound of the heart that can pull us back into the past and leave us wishing that we could change things. An important question Lovers must ask is this: *Can I love my own regret as an expression of how much I care?* If you didn't care, after all, you would have no regrets. So honor that feeling.

Nothing shines a light on what we value like death. At the end of most people's lives, when they look back, they tend to cherish the love they have for the people closest to them. They don't think about money or success; they think about relationships.

But if you ignore what you truly care about, regret will sink its tentacles into your sensitive heart and destroy your Lover energy. Life may even force your hand if you don't start paying attention to what matters. People you love may pass away, or you may find yourself in a situation where you almost die.

### Fear of Rejection

Many people who suffer from a deficiency in Lover energy often first experience a lack of love in childhood. Perhaps their parents or guardians didn't really see them for who they are. Perhaps they expressed emotions in an unhealthy way. Perhaps they made their love conditional, based on performance or looks. Or perhaps they didn't show compassion in difficult moments. But Lovers are naturally very sensitive to rejection, avoidance, coldness, or anger. So what may seem like a minor slight to some may be intense for those with insufficient Lover energy to handle it.

When we don't receive enough love in our lives, we can sometimes sour and turn dark. And Lover energy turned dark is one of the most dangerous energies in the world. We all know the stories of brutal dictators, terrorists, or mass shooters who were neglected and lacked love as children and ended up trafficking in rage and hate. Lover energy, when it transitions from deficiency into darkness, can become the most destructive force in the world.

To heal this deficiency in the soul of humankind, we must all live up to our true Lover potential and share our compassion with those who need it the most. It's easy to love those who are well off. The question is whether we, as a species, can love our broken brothers and sisters and nurture them back into balance. That will be the ultimate test of the human spirit over the next generation.

### Lack of Validation

It's not uncommon for a Lover in deficit to have experienced invalidation, shame, or guilt early in life. Abuse, neglect, violence, and loss or rejection can all lead to a shrinking of the heart. A lack of self-worth or self-love is often at the core of deficient Lover energy.

When people feel insecure and invalidated around their body image, their mental acuity, their financial situation, their relationships, their accomplishments, or their life direction, their self-worth can quickly sink and they can find themselves in a downward spiral that convinces them they have no value. This belief is crippling to Lover energy. A lack of self-esteem can stunt growth and bury fulfillment under an avalanche of pain. I don't think it would be a stretch to say that a fair majority of people in the world today suffer from deficiency in their hearts caused by a lack of validation.

## The Lover in Excess

Many Lovers in excess have an easier time caring for other people than for themselves. Even though they may know that the key to their awakening and happiness lies in turning their love inward and finding self-worth, this can be a difficult task in practice. When Lover energy is out of balance and leaning toward excess, some have an easier time giving than receiving love. This can manifest as:

- Obsessive zeal

- Poor boundaries

- Overcommitment

- Irrationality

- Idealistic goals

- Blind trust

- The need to be a martyr

- Unrealistic hopes

- Unhealthy attachments

These characteristics are encouraged primarily by three behaviors: self-sacrifice, poor establishment and maintenance of boundaries, and energy drain.

### Self-Sacrifice

Lovers in excess tend to sacrifice their energy for the sake of others. They may also indulge in blind trust or irrationality or be intoxicated by unrealistic hopes. In excess, the heart can take over and put the rational mind in the back seat. And this can lead to a naive insistence on seeing only the best in people, and then getting hurt by their more negative tendencies.

### Poor Boundaries

Trouble establishing and maintaining boundaries is also a common trait for Lovers in excess: Mothers who give all of their time and energy to their children, not leaving any for themselves. People who put all their efforts into relationships without receiving anything in return. Spiritual leaders who sacrifice their own needs and desires for the sake of their students. CEOs who, out of love for their employees, work themselves to death to provide for them. Good friends who are overwhelmed by others' drama. The list is endless.

### Energy Drain

Lover energy in excess can untether the heart from the mind, causing it to become too idealistic. Lovers in excess give away too much energy while receiving nothing in return. And this can lead to the opposite of the intended goal. In this sense, there are many similarities between excessive Lover energy and excessive Healer energy. In fact, they are energetic first cousins. The difference is that Lovers in excess attempt to give and receive love in an imbalanced way, while Healers in excess try to fix people and situations across a broad spectrum of emotions, resulting in an unhealthy use of energy.

## Back to Balance

Life is a school for learning about love. The Lover in each of us is the part that holds intimate relationships, friendships, and family in very high regard. The Lover knows that honesty, integrity, and kindness are essential for healthy relationships. Lovers who are living their truth and are in balance understand that using people as a means to an end is intolerable to the spirit.

The heart wants wholeness. So it often seeks it in others. And that's okay; it's natural. But for Lover energy to be truly fulfilled, it must find that wholeness *in itself*, and then share it with others who also feel that wholeness in themselves. This takes work— work that most people aren't willing to do. We are *love lazy*. We sit on our couches hoping our soul mates will just show up and sweep us off our feet.

The desire to fantasize rather than actually heal and grow can be very seductive, because the fantasy in our minds makes our bodies feel better—temporarily. The hope of a fulfilling future can obscure a realization of the emptiness of the moment, and this hope can be intoxicating to the Lover in us. But it's important to acknowledge reality. If there is emptiness, we must feel it. That emptiness also needs our love.

### Meditation to Balance Lover Energy

Try this simple visualization to bring your Lover energy into balance so you can manifest it in your life.

**Step 1:** With your eyes closed and your body relaxed, draw your energy and attention inward. Say hello to your inner Lover. Imagine holding a beautiful golden flower in your hand with the word "hello" written on it. Send the flower right into your heart center in the middle of your chest. Feel the hello.

**Step 2:** Ask your inner Lover what quality of energy it most wants to cultivate and express into the world. Compassion? Acceptance? Honesty? Authenticity? Love? Joy? Bliss? Or something else? Allow yourself to choose one energy for the moment.

**Step 3:** How would you feel and what would your actions look like if you mastered this energy and truly harnessed it?

**Step 4:** Allow yourself to have more of this energy. Feel it in your body with the awareness that you are ready to cultivate it and share it with the world. Every energy has a certain frequency to it—a kind of vibration. Feel that energy in your body and allow it to radiate around you.

**Step 5:** Notice that cultivating this energy and sharing it with the world are actually part of your soul's purpose in life. Without cultivating it, you may never truly find what you are looking for. Recognize this important life lesson and mission.

**Step 6:** See an image in your mind's eye of what your life will look like as you truly harness this energy. How will the people around you respond and feel? How will you live your life differently?

**Step 7:** Feel your inner Lover; truly own this energy and find balance in your heart. Recognize that you are a Lover in the true sense of the word, and that being a Lover is part of your soul's gift to you and to everyone on this planet.

## Lover Self-Reflection

Follow up this meditation with self-reflection. Ask yourself these questions to help you identify your deficient Lover tendencies:

- Do you feel a consistent lack of self-worth or self-love?

- Do you have a hard time listening to your heart and being authentic?

- Do you tend to have trouble establishing boundaries and give more than you receive?

- Do you have a hard time trusting and building deep relationships?

- Do you avoid relationships in order to avoid pain or disappointment?

Now ask yourself these questions to help you identify your excessive Lover tendencies:

- Do you have an easier time giving than receiving?

- Do you find yourself overly willing to sacrifice yourself for the sake of others?

- Do you tend to trust people blindly and end up getting hurt?

- Do you often have trouble with unhealthy attachments and relationships?

- Are you too idealistic? Do you avoid the realities of the world?

Finally, consider these questions as you work to cultivate balanced Lover energy:

- Do I generally feel that my heart is open to the world or closed?

- When I make important decisions, do I consult my heart?

- Do I feel as if I give more, receive more, or give and receive love equally?

- Am I willing to face any pain in my heart in order to heal and open to the world?

- If I were living up to my full Lover potential, how would I show up differently in the world?

### Lover Goals

Consider the difference between how Lover energy works internally and externally. See if you can come up with three ways in which you can apply your Lover energy to your life on an internal level. For example:

- Exhibit more self-acceptance and self-love.

- Release past relationship pain.

- Be more honest with myself.

Now write down three ways in which you can apply your Lover energy to your life on an external level. For example:

- Communicate my needs better.

- Give time and resources to my favorite nonprofit.

- Take good care of my family.

### Lover Action: Loving-Kindness

Buddhist tradition employs a meditation called *metta* to promote loving-kindness. The power behind the meditation lies in cultivating the energetic light of love within yourself and then radiating that light out beyond yourself in greater and greater circles. The goal of the practice is eventually to encompass whole cities or even the whole world in love and compassion.

This exercise is similar to the Buddhist practice, but involves a series of actions designed to express Lover energy out into the world in a manifested way.

First, spend some time writing a short love letter to yourself in your journal. This may sound silly—and it may feel silly when you're doing it. It may also be a lot harder to do than you think. If that is the case, it is a sign of deficient Lover energy within you. If it takes longer to write the letter than you originally planned, return to the task until the letter is complete. But try to make the letter at least one whole page in length.

Write the letter as though you were telling a close friend or partner how much you care about them and why. List the things you are grateful for in yourself. Once you are finished, write down one thing, one gift, you'd like to give yourself. It can be something small—perhaps a cup of coffee or a bouquet of flowers that you might not otherwise have "splurged" on. But it can also be something intangible or emotionally charged. For example, what if you took a whole day off from criticizing yourself?

Now extend that gift outward. What can you do this week to give a gift of loving-kindness to a friend or family member? This doesn't have to be a physical gift. Consider cleaning the kitchen on a night when it isn't your turn or cooking a special meal for your partner. Call up a friend you haven't contacted in a while.

Now extend that gift outward again. How can you show loving-kindness to strangers in your community? Can you smile more at people while making your way through your day? Let service workers know that you appreciate what they do? This may sound obvious, or even a little bit clichéd, but these small and seemingly insignificant moments can very often make a huge difference for others.

The final stage of the practice is probably the most difficult. Consider ways in which you can show this same loving-kindness, this same Lover energy, to those you don't particularly like or perhaps even resent. Don't feel that you have to rush to forgive major injustices right away. Just consider what it might mean to let go of a minor resentment or grudge. You don't have to reestablish ties with anyone or reach out to someone you've removed from your life. But if you can release some of your emotional attachment to that hurt and allow some forgiveness to take its place, you will have made more room for Lover energy in your life.

# Chapter 7

# The Artist

*Art enables us to find ourselves and
lose ourselves at the same time.*
—Thomas Merton

Awakening Artist energy pulls inspiration down
from the heavens and up from the earth, makes the
unseen seen, and gives the emotional present form
in the material world through the vehicle of creative expression. Artist energy transports us out of
the realm of our regrets and anxieties. It illuminates
the present moment by evoking an intuitive, visceral,
emotional response. The Artist is inherently a master
of both process and presence.

When Artist energy really begins to reach its
potential in you, it doesn't do so for money, or fame,
or fortune. It does so for the experience of the *process*.
Artist energy is the conduit, the medium, for universal creativity. As the Artist in you flowers, you may
begin to recognize that perhaps the deepest reason

for creation is the sheer joy of the work. The means, in this case, *is* the end. For the Artist, it's all about the *creating*, and not about the *creation*.

Artist energy is also a force for the present. It gives our ego-centered minds, which are constantly thinking about the future and the past, a rest in this divine moment. And it doesn't matter whether the person is creating the art or experiencing it; both are invited into this moment.

Have you ever found yourself totally dissolved in the here and now without a care in the world when lost in a book, a song, or a dance or when laughing uncontrollably at some comedy? Artist energy is what pulls us into this presence and helps us recognize the sacredness of the moment, through beauty and perspective. It gives the invisible form so that we can enjoy other dimensions through our human experience.

Artist energy also cultivates freedom in the human spirit and pulls it out of darkness. During the Renaissance, art, music, and culture all flowered, and a new age of science was born as the restrictions of the old ways began to be challenged. Michelangelo and Leonardo da Vinci changed our perspective on the world through their art and science. They and their contemporaries paved the way for philosophers like René Descartes and Baruch Spinoza, challenging us with new ways of looking at the world. Explorers like Galileo Galilei and Isaac Newton rode the wave of the Renaissance and moved humanity forward more quickly in 100 years than it had moved in the previous 1,000.

And this is part of the purpose of Artist energy—to push back against common paradigms and worldviews. The Artist works to share and shape perspective. The power of Artist energy lies in its ability to open the mind and heart to new possibilities—to alternate dimensions and to an appreciation of diversity.

## The Artist in Balance

Art can heal people and provide hope in unexpected ways. A friend told me about a man from London who had been in prison for fourteen years in Guantanamo Bay in Cuba on charges of terrorism. The man was innocent, but he nonetheless spent a substantial portion of his life in a prison cell. The guards tried to torture him day after day by blasting him with rock music. They played one song in particular—while the music itself was loud, the lyrics were essentially hopeful and uplifting. He repeated the lyrics over and over to himself which gave him the strength to continue living until he was eventually released. So instead of hurting him as they intended, the song actually gave him hope. It helped him get through the difficult days.

The music freed him spiritually from the intense physical confinement he was experiencing. And although this story is extreme, it's not unique. Art, in whatever form it takes, frees us, opens our hearts and minds, and gets us through difficult times.

Balanced Artist energy is a powerful force for creation, invention, and innovation. Those who enjoy it are:

- Creative

- Imaginative

- Open-minded

- Appreciative of beauty

- Able to flow with life

- Self-validating

- Expressive

- Original

- Authentic

- Sensitive

- Work to change paradigms

- Embrace hobbies and play

If you take a deep look inside yourself, you may not find a rock star or a Picasso, but you *will* find your own inner Artist. And that Artist, if awakened to its full potential, may have a profound effect on the world.

The trick to mastering life and being fulfilled is to become the most "you" that you can be. Artist energy, as you master and express it, awakens your authentic self to the world. It helps you become comfortable with your creativity and with being seen. Artist energy is the vehicle for universal creativity and expression. Unlocking its potential in you may be a deep part of your journey through life.

## The Artist in Deficit

When your Artist energy is deficient, you may have a hard time validating your creativity or letting yourself be seen. It may be difficult for you to express who you really are to the world or to complete creative projects. It may be challenging for you to see the world from different perspectives.

Characteristics that are common in those who have deficient Artist energy include:

- Avoiding true passion

- Not valuing creativity

- Allowing criticism to thwart creativity

- Believing in limiting thoughts

- Overwhelming self-judgment

- Being paralyzed by invalidation

- Being incapacitated by fear of failure

- Apathy

- Lack of imagination

- Lack of a clear vision

- Disconnection from deeper levels of life

- Excessive practicality

Most people who aren't professional Artists underestimate the power of this energy and don't realize how much balance, happiness, and fulfillment they can bring to their lives by unleashing it. They see "art" as an extracurricular activity, a nonessential luxury. Artists in deficit often don't recognize that art is as essential to life as all the other energies.

There are three main traits that tend to suppress Artist energy: low self-esteem, fear of judgment, and an inability to bring projects or plans to completion.

### Low Self-Esteem

Artist energy often gets invalidated at an early age. We are taught to believe that we aren't talented enough, and so we never try. This lack of validation can also lead to apathy and depression if we don't let our hearts sing.

Low self-esteem can also trap us into a compulsion to make comparisons. Constantly comparing our creations to those of others can lead to deep invalidating feelings that paralyze our creativity. We often only see other people's completed, edited, or smoothly sanded creations. Then we compare these to our lump of clay or our book in progress, and the difference stops us in our tracks. But how long and how much work did it take for those finished works to rise to that level of excellence? I can guarantee it didn't happen overnight—in fact, it probably happened over thousands of nights.

### Fear of Judgment

Another common sign of a deficiency in Artist energy is a fear of judgment. Why try if I'm just going to be criticized? But judgment is an unavoidable challenge that the Artist must face in order to grow. The silver lining comes when we learn to take healthy input that can make us better and allow destructive criticism to pass through us.

Artists weather the storms of judgment by practicing loving self-kindness. They come to know that their own true value isn't based on what others think. Of course, we all understand that intellectually. But truly *knowing* it and *living* it require that we create art and share it with the world. They require that we let ourselves be seen, experience negative feedback, and continue creating anyway—over and over again.

### The Land of Half-Finished Projects

Perhaps the place where Artists get stuck more than anywhere else is what I call the "land of half-finished projects." Envision a junkyard of incomplete sentences, of unfinished songs, of half-done paintings, of jokes with premises but no punch lines, of stories without endings. This is the wasteland that the Artist must avoid. As Artists, we must be vigilant to avoid making excuses about why we can't follow our intentions through to the very end.

Nothing creates certainty and bolsters Artist energy more than finishing something. The Artist's mantra should be: Finish. Finish. Finish.

## The Artist in Excess

The freedom and creativity that Artist energy harnesses must be balanced in order to flower fully. When this energy is in excess, the lower unresolved energies of the individual ego may gain the upper hand. History is littered with examples of Artists who lived lives of addiction or who overdosed, who failed in countless relationships, and who suffered from narcissism or loneliness.

Dangers for the Artist in excess include:

- Perfectionism

- Overcompetitiveness

- Constant comparisons to others

- Ungrounded or out-of-body experiences

- Hardened point of view

- Excessive need to be seen

- Extreme idealism

- Impractical mindset

- Pride in going against the mainstream

- Obsession with creativity

- An insatiable need for validation

- Difficulty receiving input

- A my-way-or-the-highway mentality

- A poor relationship with money

- Too much fantasizing

The four main pitfalls that contribute to an excess in Artist energy are unrealistic standards, an obsession with purity, a controlling ego, and that familiar enemy—perfectionism.

### Unrealistic Standards

The Artist energy in us can often be guilty of wanting the world to be in color when it comes to expression but in black and white when it comes to values. Artists tend to have very high standards and can suffer from an all-or-nothing mentality. This can lead to an inability to compromise: *I won't do corporate. I won't work with children. I'm not interested in making something commercial or useful.*

### Obsession with Purity

Those who fail to control an excess of Artist energy can fall prey to such a love for purity that it can lead to great pain and isolation. They may seem impractical in their approach to life and not very understanding of people who don't share their point of view. They may disdain the need to have a "regular" job or steady income and borrow large amounts of money from family and friends, not recognizing that their idealism is straining their relationships with the people they love.

### Controlling Ego

Excess Artist energy can also manifest as an inflation of the ego. The praise that a successful Artist receives can be pretty overwhelming for the fragile human psyche to handle. When Artists go from zero to hero in the eyes of the world, they can quickly begin to identify their self-worth with their creations. And this, indeed, is a double-edged sword for all the essential energies. We've all watched what happens to actors, writers, comedians, or musicians who find fame and fortune, only to be undone by their dreams coming true because they are unable to handle the maddening attention and high expectations.

True Artist energy, whether amateur or professional, reaches its highest potential when the ego gets out of the way. The experience of "no-self"—of there being nothing but the music, the art, the dance—is the place where Artists can lose themselves in the moment, in the act. It is where Artists break from their inner dialogue and critic. And this is the ultimate gift of Artist energy.

### Perfectionism

Artists must be very vigilant to control their need for perfection. Perfectionism can be the ultimate seduction for the Artist in excess, because it burns out Artist energy. Although this same dynamic plays out in many energies in your life, it's particularly poison-ous for Artists, because Artist energy is about expression and creativity, not control. When Artist energy loses balance and falls into excess, however, it begins objectifying the moment and the art for future gain.

## Back to Balance

Elizabeth Gilbert, author of *Eat, Pray, Love*, gave a wonderful TED Talk in which she described how she had to face the probability that her most celebrated work was behind her. She described having to grapple with the intense public expectations that have led many authors to alcoholism and depression. She went on to explain how the ancient Greeks and Romans had dealt with this problem. They simply credited their creativity to inspiring entities called *daimons* (Greek) and *genii* (Roman) who were not creatives themselves, but rather vehicles of divine inspiration. This took the onus off the Artist and placed it firmly in the realm of magic. The value of art came to reside in the process, in the moment, rather than in the product. And this is where it resides for those who have achieved true balance in their Artist energy.

### *Meditation to Balance Artist Energy*

As you work through this meditation, consider how you can bring more of an awareness of the artistic process and the present moment into your day-to-day life.

**Step 1:** Begin by acknowledging your inner Artist energy. Now that you have grounded some other deficient and excessive energies, focus on tapping into your inner Artist's ability to have creative vision. Explore what creative vision in you is ready to be born.

**Step 2:** Imagine yourself sitting in a room in the center of your head. In front of you, there is a large movie screen showing the night sky shimmering with twinkling stars.

**Step 3:** Begin to notice that there is a new star being born right in front of your eyes. It gets closer and closer to you. The light of this star begins to project an image out in front of you, the way the light from a movie projector casts images onto a screen.

**Step 4:** This image is no ordinary image, however. It is a deeply creative vision of something your inner Artist is here to fulfill. It may be art, music, writing, dancing, or some other creative endeavor.

**Step 5:** If you have a hard time seeing the vision, try bringing it closer to you or moving it back. It may need a moment to load and then come into focus. What does this vision show you? If you had no limitations on your creativity, what would want to be born out of your inner Artist?

**Step 6:** Allow yourself to feel this vision. Notice the truth, the power, the energy in it. Does it want to be born for the sake of creativity? To heal? To connect? To enlighten others? What is the purpose of this creation? And are you ready to commit to birthing it?

**Step 7:** As you own this vision, begin to validate and own your inner Artist. It's been waiting long enough. Give yourself and the world the gift of this vision. And when you step out of this meditation, take your first or next step toward creating it.

As soon as you can after you complete your meditation, take a few minutes to journal what your vision was and how you can commit to it. This doesn't have to be a vision to paint the next Sistine Chapel ceiling or write the next award-winning novel. It may simply be a vision of writing twenty minutes every morning.

### Artist Self-Reflection

To make this meditation more powerful, follow up with some careful self-reflection. To identify your deficient Artist tendencies, ask yourself these questions:

- Do you often find yourself feeling invalidated or afraid of being creative?

- Do you feel limitations around pursuing your artistic passions?

- Do you dim your light down to avoid your creations being criticized?

- Do you allow others to shape your paradigm of the world excessively?

Now ask yourself these questions to help identify your excessive Artist tendencies:

- Do you often find yourself lost in fantasy?

- Do you tend to be overly idealistic in your worldview?

- Do you have a hard time grounding your creations in a successful career?

- Do you go overboard with your creativity
  and need everything to come out perfectly
  every time?

- Are you in resistance to the practicalities of
  the physical world?

Finally, consider these questions as you work to cultivate balanced Artist energy:

- Do I allow myself to be playful, and how
  does that show up in my life?

- If time, money, and responsibilities were not
  factors, how would I use my Artist energy
  on a daily basis?

- What other activities could I give up if
  I wanted to practice art on a daily basis?
  How?

- What people do I admire in my life who
  use their Artist energy in a healthy way?
  How can I engage them and show them my
  admiration?

### Artist Goals

Consider the difference between how Artist energy works internally and externally. Then see if you can come up with three ways in which you can apply your Artist energy to your life on an internal level. For example:

- Give myself permission to be creative.

- Be more open to playfulness.

- Appreciate my unique perspective.

Now write down three ways in which you can apply your Artist energy to your life on an external level. For example:

- Take a painting, drawing, pottery, acting, or writing class.

- Design my home space.

- Bring more creativity into my career.

### Artist Action: Intuitive Play

The obvious activity here is to create art! If you have never tried to create a piece of art—whether it's writing a poem, painting a still life, drawing a portrait, singing, or playing an instrument—I encourage you to take that first step. This first step can sometimes be the hardest part of the act of creation—staring at that blank paper, that empty computer file, or that bare canvas—so experiment with intuitive art for a while to get yourself out of that perfectionist headspace. Scribble, splash paint, slap words together that make no sense, make lists of favorite words, play random notes, or make up weird songs and sing them to your cat.

For example, take out a piece of paper right now and a pen or some crayons. Don't stress too much over having the "right" materials—a piece of printer paper or even a piece of lined notebook paper is fine. And if all you have is a pencil or a ballpoint pen, perfect. You'd be amazed at what some Artists have accomplished with just these basic tools after they've put in the time, process, and practice. If you want to draw something in front of you, go for it. Otherwise just start scribbling.

After a while, you may notice shapes and lines in conversation with each other on the page, or you may become fascinated by what's created on the page every time one line intersects with another. You may even find that, after a while, you reach a headspace similar to the one you get to in meditation. That's because, while your hands and mind are occupied with drawing, your soul is free to rest, to find flow, and to achieve peace.

Remember that, while I do emphasize the need to finish a work, this doesn't mean that you must always create "good" work. The point is the process and the presence. When you are finished with a piece, be proud of the work you put into it, even if you believe it's not "good." This is, after all, utterly subjective. There is a lot of art in the world, and for every piece of art there are people who love it and people who hate it. (No matter what it is or who the author is—I promise you.) Be proud that you started it, be glad that you worked on it, and feel satisfied when you declare it finished.

You are an Artist! Go out and buy yourself some sidewalk chalk or a box of crayons or some other playful tools to exercise your unique Artist energy.

# Chapter 8

# The Explorer

*The most beautiful thing we can experience is the mysterious. It is the source of all true art and science. He to whom the emotion is a stranger, who can no longer pause to wonder and stand wrapped in awe, is as good as dead; his eyes are closed.*

—Albert Einstein

We are a deeply curious species. We all have an innate desire to experience the mysterious. This is Explorer energy. It's the feeling, the need, the subtle intuition in each of us to go to the edge and beyond. To open, unfold, and see. To discover, uncover, and know. Explorers want to experience the unknown and, ultimately, are much less interested in the destination than in the journey.

The Explorer in you may be attracted to travel, to seeing into the farthest reaches of space, to understanding the workings of the human body on a cellular level, or to reaching back into history to ascertain the reasons why civilizations developed in certain directions. Scientists, astronauts, adventurers, and anthropologists all have this in common. They need to understand and explore.

Explorers may be intellectual in nature, like academic researchers, or focused on the physical, like scuba divers or hikers. One commonality among those who are working on manifesting their inner Explorer energy is that they yearn for the "beyond." If they had been born on a different planet in a different galaxy, their souls would still desire to see past the horizons of their world.

The external world may seem infinite to Explorers. And, in fact, it *becomes* infinite when they close their physical eyes and open their inner eye. Some explore these inner worlds through meditation, intuitive perception, and consciousness. Others like to see into the dimensions of the human psyche. Inside each of us, in the depths of our being, there is so much to be explored.

Children naturally embody the energy of openness, wonder, and curiosity. When I was five or six years old, I spent hours staring at ants, watching them build their civilization by moving grains of sand and dead bugs from one place to another, losing myself in their world. You probably had similar experiences as a child. Perhaps you stared at every part of a flower, memorizing its color and shape. Or maybe you chased lightning bugs or peered up into the stars in wonder, captivated by the sheer magnitude of the night sky. And the part of you that, as a child, wanted to know why a leaf is green or why the stars shine is still within you, waiting to resurface in your consciousness.

There is no one right way to be an Explorer. Society may hold scientists in higher esteem than children looking at bugs, but both are a manifestation of Explorer energy. I once had the incredible opportunity of participating in a group discussion on the topic of curiosity at the MIT Center for Bits and Atoms. It was led by a brilliant physicist who shared this story. A young boy once asked him: "We know the speed of light, but what is the speed of darkness?" This physicist, who was at the top of his game at the time, had never thought of exploring the speed of darkness. At that moment, however, he was struck by how important the question was. And he realized how incredibly perceptive children can be.

Unfortunately, adults can be too predictable. We act from habit. We trade spontaneity for certainty. We sacrifice our sense of wonder for our need for security and control. When we do that over time, our Explorer energy goes dormant and life loses some of its meaning. We become disconnected from the wonder of space and the planets. We dim the stars with artificial light and cover the ground with cement.

We move in a kind of two-dimensional, horizontal world—looking forward and back, but never up and down. We forget that we live in an infinite universe and complain about the little things that bother us.

As Explorers peel back each layer of life, they sit in awe of the complexity, the simplicity, and the beauty of life's infinite forms. The curiosity and sense of wonder they have when they confront the sheer magnificence of life are an almost spiritual experience for them—something that puts them in touch with the purpose and meaning of existence. For Explorers, the *why* of life is not a question to be answered; it is a path to be experienced.

## The Explorer in Balance

Explorers are living up to their potential when they understand that life is what happens while we are making other plans. Explorer energy teaches us to connect with the pulse of life, with the current of the river of life. It helps us let go of the resistance that clogs the pipes through which the energy of curiosity and discovery flows.

Explorers in balance are:

- Curious

- Enthusiastic

- Dreamers

- Thirsty for knowledge

- Joyful in new experiences

- Energetic travelers

- Deeply appreciative of the mysteries of life

- Open-minded

- Curious about how things work

- Perceptive

- Trailblazers

Explorers in balance are the conduits through which our innate powers of discovery flow out into the wider world.

Lovers are energized by giving and receiving love, while Creators are energized by building things of value. But Explorers thrive on the journey through life itself. I have traveled a fair amount in my life, exploring this beautiful planet. I once spent forty-five hours traveling across India on a train, from Delhi to Chennai, sitting in the second-class unair-conditioned compartment. If I had been going to a job, or a funeral, or some unhappy event, I probably would have arrived exhausted. But the Explorer in me was so excited by the journey that I arrived full of energy.

As I matured into a teacher, I began leading retreats, taking groups to places like Costa Rica, Bali, and Bhutan, because I recognized that what made me happy was awakening the Explorer in others. The Lover, the Explorer, and the Master in me combined to inspire me to share my experiences and my insights with others. To this day, almost nothing makes me happier than seeing the faces of those approaching the Himalayas for the first time, then sitting them down to meditate and allowing the mountains to teach them.

Explorers in balance can tap into a deep well of enthusiasm and stamina when they find the right path. And, for them, finding their way is part of the journey. Explorers in balance are trailblazers who chart new and original directions. Or they may travel paths that have been trod before, but see them with new eyes and a fresh perspective. However they move forward, they need energy and fuel for their journey. And they find that energy and fuel in enthusiasm and wonder. You have to find that inspiration in yourself and light your own fire.

## The Explorer in Deficit

Explorers in deficit lack the fuel to ignite their curiosity and wonder. Some are inherently homebodies. Some don't like to travel; some have no interest in science or space. These people may believe they don't have an inner Explorer. But perhaps they simply haven't validated the part of themselves that loves to read history, study anthropology, understand other cultures and languages, or even just peer into an anthill or contemplate a flower. These are all activities that use Explorer energy. And when that energy is in deficit, it can be difficult to strike out in new directions.

Deficient Explorer energy manifests as:

- Anxiety and fear of the unknown

- A belief in false limitations

- Avoidance of adventure

- Acceptance of assumptions without questioning them

- Excessive concern for safety

- A tendency to devalue discovery and mystery

- A belief that everything has already been figured out

- A lack of imagination and wonder

- Lack of interest in the unknown

- Lack of curiosity about how things work

The three traits that contribute most to deficient Explorer energy are self-limitation, apathy and disinterest, and paralyzing fear.

### Self-Limitation

The Explorer's great nemesis is self-limitation. Of course, when cultivating Explorer energy, you must understand your *external* limitations so you can break through them when necessary. Scientists, for instance, may be limited by a lack of funding or technological capability. Travelers may have to contend with closed borders or insufficient time or money. Astronauts may be challenged by the incalculable distances that put certain stars out of reach. But you must also recognize and conquer your self-imposed *internal* limitations. One of the greatest obstacles—and one of the greatest opportunities—for Explorers is to understand their own self-generated limiting beliefs.

If the greatest strength of Explorers is their ability to move into the unknown, their greatest weakness lies in believing in false limitations that deny the possibility of making the journey. Moreover, as you rise to your own potential in this area of life, you will be challenged, not only by your own limitations and fears, but by other people's as well. The greatest danger for Explorers is the temptation to surrender to others' lack of vision, their fears, and the sense of invalidation that colors their view of life.

### Apathy and Disinterest

Explorers in deficit may also find themselves avoiding the journey due to apathy. But to avoid the journey through apathy and disinterest is to miss out on something very sacred. To be born with eyes to see, but to choose to keep them closed is to miss out on the mystery of life. When we succumb to apathy and lose interest in the journey, it is nothing less than a tragedy for the soul.

Those with deficient Explorer energy may find themselves never leaving the place in which they grew up. They may avoid new experiences by relying on repetition and habit, playing video games, or vicariously participating in the adventures of others through television or social media. They may never pursue anything new themselves.

When in deficit, Explorers may cling to excuses and amplify those excuses in order to avoid real experiences. They may become chronic complainers, always ready to see and point out the negative in life, shielding themselves from the new or the unknown. They may remain indifferent to what's over the next hill. Explorers in deficit may lack gratitude for the majesty of life.

### Paralyzing Fear

If realizing the potential of Explorer energy means reaching out to the new and the unknown, then its deficiency means shying away from new experiences out of fear. In fact, fear is the paralyzing force that stops Explorers dead in their tracks—fear of the unknown, fear of failure, fear of what other people think, fear of not being smart enough, fear of taking the wrong path. To remain in balance, Explorers must learn to differentiate between useful fears that can serve to protect them and destructive fear that is meant to be conquered.

Overcoming fear, whether you are a rock climber or a blogger sharing your first travel post with the world, gives you energy. It firms up the path on which you walk. It deepens you as a person. It takes you from living in your head to living in the world. You didn't read about the sharks, you swam with them. You didn't read about an African safari, you went on one.

What's truly important for Explorers is not the distance traveled, but the pleasure of the experience, the shift of energy, the growth that occurs along the way. How many mountains of fear, invalidation, and uncertainty have you climbed? That is the true test of the Explorer. And how much have you enjoyed it?

## The Explorer in Excess

Explorers become unbalanced and move into excess when they use the journey, the search, as an escape from themselves or from responsibility. Compulsive travelers may find themselves avoiding deep relationships or commitment to work. They may uproot themselves and take off on their next adventure just as circumstances in their lives are "getting real." Scientists may become workaholics and lose themselves in research to avoid family drama. Historians or futurists may disregard the present moment and focus too much on the lives of people long deceased or a future yet to be born.

Excess Explorer energy manifests as:

- An incessant need for more and different experiences

- Fear of missing out

- Exploring to avoid responsibility

- Disdain for the "normal" life

- Looking down on the less experienced

- Being easily bored

- Being prone to addiction

- Leaving the body too often

- Difficulty being content in the moment

Any of these traits may indicate an excess of Explorer energy. Two major causes of this imbalance are a disdain for normalcy and a weakness for what I call "rabbit holes."

### Disdain for Normalcy

A life of adventure and discovery is tantalizing—much more fun than leading a nine-to-five existence, paying the bills, and doing the laundry. But the inherent appeal of the Explorer's life can be a trap as well. When I was in my early and mid-twenties, I traveled and lived abroad for a number of years. It became a way of life for me. I lived out of my backpack in developing countries because life was easy and cheap and I didn't have to work. But after a while, I noticed I was becoming resistant to the "normal" life. I had developed disdain for living in the United States and holding down a job. I was obsessed with a certain kind of freedom that came with travel and lack of responsibility. Eventually, I realized I was actually avoiding something deep inside myself and using travel as an excuse. Explorers must learn to stay grounded in the "normal" in order to stay in balance.

### Rabbit Holes

Explorers can also lose balance by becoming overly focused on discovery—spending excessive amounts of time researching things online, reading countless books, going down "rabbit holes" looking for information on specific topics or perhaps even exploring other people's lives through social media—checking out what they are doing each day, finding out how they see the world, or discovering what makes their lives so great. The content of these inquiries doesn't matter. What matters is that the act of exploration becomes disproportionate and throws the energy out of balance.

This can extend to spiritual quests as well. When Explorers lose balance and fall into excess, even normally healthy levels of spiritual exploration can turn into avoidance and escape. Those who explore a number of mind-altering ceremonies and plants may negatively impact their health, diminish their ability to function in daily life, or sacrifice their personal relationships. What began as a search for meaning can develop into a means to escape daily responsibilities, difficult conversations, and the challenges of life.

## Back to Balance

Balanced Explorers don't travel aimlessly in the dark; they light the path of life with their intuitive awareness. This awareness, this sense, is something you develop by getting in touch with yourself through experience and meditation. If you don't test your intuition by taking chances and pulling on the invisible thread that guides you, you may end up enmeshed in the worst tragedy of all—an unlived and unexplored life.

I arrived in Hawaii in my mid-twenties with a few hundred dollars in my bank account and no place to live. I was going to study the intuitive and healing arts at a special school for mysticism that someone in India had told me about. But I had no plan, no money, and nowhere to sleep. I literally hitchhiked out of the airport, slept on someone's floor for a few weeks, and then lived in a tent for three months.

I found a job on a farm picking lettuce and another renting kayaks. There was so much uncertainty in my life at the time, but I remember making a conscious decision every day to keep following my intuitive sense that this was my path. I was meant to be at an intuitive school. Yes, I get the irony.

Most people think that Hawaii is just paradise, but when you have no money and you're alone, even paradise can suck. The only thing that kept me going on this journey was a deep knowingness in my heart that there was something I needed to learn from this school, and from the island.

I ended up spending seven years in Hawaii, eventually becoming the director of the school and building a career based on my training. When I look back at the chances I took and the shoestring budget on which I lived, I realize that, from the outside, my decision may have seemed dangerous and irrational. It also wasn't easy telling my parents, who had spent a lot of money sending me to college: "Mom, Dad, I'm moving to Hawaii to study magic!"

### Meditation to Balance Explorer Energy

The need to know how life will turn out can sometimes be born of a fear of the unknown. But to awaken your inner Explorer, you must be willing to take a journey and step out of the comfort of your own beliefs and patterns. This meditation can help.

**Step 1:** Draw your awareness inward as you close your eyes, with the intention of going on an inner journey. Recognize that, although the outer world seems bigger than the inner world, perhaps there is just as much space inside you as there is outside you. Allow yourself to be in awe of the mystery of the space, the consciousness in your body. Recognize that this space nurtures you in an indefinable way.

**Step 2:** To bring your Explorer energy back into balance and fulfill its potential, you must first be honest with who you are at a very deep level. You are an Explorer. What direction does your inner Explorer want to take? Every Explorer must choose a direction. Are you an Explorer of nature? Of space? Of the human body? Of consciousness? For now, choose one area for your focus.

**Step 3:** Ask yourself if you are truly ready to embrace the depth of this purpose in you. To help clarify this mission, think of those in your life or in human history who truly embrace Explorer energy and fulfill that part of themselves. What quality of energy do you appreciate in them? Is it curiosity? Open-mindedness? Courage? A sense of adventure?

**Step 4:** Can you see that quality in yourself and begin to embrace it? Can you notice how that quality, if fully embraced, can help you on your path as an Explorer?

**Step 5:** Has something been keeping you from embracing this quality in yourself? Can you be honest with what it is and begin to shift your energy? You do that by letting go of any excuses and fears and knowing deeply that owning this part of your energy will help you fulfill your life's purpose.

**Step 6:** Recognize that this is the beginning of the next chapter of your story. You get to write it; you get to choose and decide. Are you ready to move forward with enthusiasm and courage? Are you ready to step out into the world unapologetically? Are you ready to be the Explorer you are meant to be?

**Step 7:** Bring your Explorer back into balance, validate it, and see your next step in your mind's eye. This is your journey, and it's time for your inner Explorer to come fully into its own.

As you finish your meditation, take time to jot down your thoughts and feelings in your journal. How does your body feel right now? Are you motivated or energized? What would you like to do next?

### Explorer Self-Reflection

As always, meditation is more effective when followed by self-reflection. Ask yourself these questions to help identify your deficient Explorer tendencies:

- Do you tend to be afraid of the unknown?

- Do you forget to look up at the stars or explore what lies beneath your feet?

- Have you lost your sense of adventure?

- Has your innate curiosity been invalidated in some way?

- Do you forget how important it is to explore both the inner and outer world?

Now ask yourself these questions to help identify your excessive Explorer tendencies:

- Do you tend to lose yourself in exploration to avoid the mundane parts of life?

- Do you often experience the fear of missing out?

- Are you addicted to adventure?

- Do you feel as if you always need to figure out how everything works?

- Do you frequently ignore your family and friends for new people, new adventures?

Finally, consider these questions as you begin to cultivate balanced Explorer energy:

- In what ways in my life have responsibility and day-to-day tasks covered up my curious inner Explorer?

- How can I change those tasks so they make me notice more?

- What people do I look up to in my life who truly embody Explorer energy? How can I engage them to learn about their work or how they see the world?

### Explorer Goals

Consider the difference between how Explorer energy works internally and externally. Then see if you can come up with three ways in which you can apply your Explorer energy to your life on an internal level. For example:

- Have more courage to explore.

- Be comfortable with uncertainty.

- Explore my inner space.

Now write down three ways in which you can apply your Explorer energy to your life on an external level. For example:

- Travel around the world.

- Take an astronomy course.

- Go for a long hike.

### Explorer Action: Adventure Retreat

The best way to balance and replenish your Explorer energy is to indulge your curiosity. Try new things!

Go on an adventure! And, while world travel is exciting, you don't have to fly to distant lands to find adventure. We sometimes get so bogged down in our own small worlds and restrictive patterns that we forget that there is an enormous amount of adventure to be found right outside our doors, in our own cities, or counties, or states.

Chances are that there are areas close to where you live that you haven't explored. All this exercise really entails is that you set aside a day and go explore them. Perhaps a local park or nature preserve. Perhaps a part of town you've not visited before. Or perhaps a nearby city. Take along a friend and make a day of it. Try new food; seek out new experiences; see new things! You may want to plan certain parts of your day, of course, and looking at maps can be part of the experience. And naturally, you'll want to make sure you are prepared and safe on your adventure. But be sure to allow some room for spontaneity. Make occasional intuitive choices and open yourself up to the possibility of getting a little lost.

Life is inexhaustible! There is no end to what is possible. But that shouldn't dissuade the Explorer in you from striking out in new directions. It should excite you. Learn to enjoy the ride, and the Explorer in you will awaken to this boundless adventure we call life.

# Chapter 9

# The Master

*We shall not cease from exploration*
*And the end of all our exploring*
*Will be to arrive where we started*
*And know the place for the first time.*

—T. S. Eliot

The Master is the seeker of truth. It's the part of you that searches for self-realization through introspection, understanding, and wisdom. Master energy drives your desire to share that light with the world. This is the part of you that knows that the journey isn't ultimately about arriving *someplace else*; it's about arriving *here*, in this moment, into your own being. In the Master, you recognize your true nature behind all of the forms that the other energies of your soul have taken.

People who awaken their true inner Master may use that energy to become teachers, writers, healers, or guides. Or they may stay hidden from society and only affect the world more subtly. Those who have reached their spiritual potential are not necessarily drawn to any specific vocation, and there's no predicting what direction the energy of an awakened Master will take. I've heard singers reach notes that were so divine that everyone in the audience found themselves touching very high states of spirituality. I've read writers who channeled the most eloquent poetry that touched the deepest parts of the human heart. Others, through their sheer presence, emanate an aura of inner peace so powerful that it transforms those around them.

No two Master energies are the same, because the lens through which the light of the soul expresses itself is always different. Spiritual masters throughout history—from the Buddha, to Jesus, to Lao Tzu, to the Dalai Lama—have all had unique personalities and teaching styles. And as you awaken and share your own inner light, you will be different as well. And that difference should be celebrated.

One of my favorite teachers is author and professor of comparative religion Joseph Campbell, who wrote *The Hero with a Thousand Faces*. The premise of this book is that there is a foundational and repeating story pattern that plays out in the lore and teachings of many religious and spiritual traditions.

Heroes, Campbell argues, live normal lives until they are unexpectedly called to an adventure that changes them forever by allowing them to confront and overcome challenges, achieve wisdom, and unlock their true potential. This archetypal narrative can be found in many myths, legends, and epic cycles, as well as in contemporary fiction and cinema, some popular examples being the *Lord of the Rings* trilogy by J. R. R. Tolkien and the *Star Wars* movies.

Campbell finds the same archetype in the world's spiritual traditions. Throughout history, stories of awakening, journeying, and transformation have taught us about Master energy and how it manifests. The Buddha, for example, was a prince living in sheltered privilege until he was faced with the realities of sickness and death. These experiences sent him on a quest that ultimately resulted in enlightenment and the sharing of that wisdom with others. Mother Teresa heard the call to help the poor and downtrodden in Kolkata, India—a call most people would have completely ignored. She answered it and taught the world the true meaning of unconditional love and compassion. And there are so many more examples.

We all possess the ability to embark on our own hero's journey. It will look different for each of us, but the possibilities for revelation and transformation are available to each of us no matter where we are in our lives. Still, many of us are afraid of being ostracized or humiliated for taking risks or for making seemingly countercultural choices. Some of us, for a variety of reasons, may never respond to the call in the first place. But for those who do, the energy of the Master, when it awakens to its potential, marks the place where we begin to perceive deep inner truths born of pure experience, not just intellect. And once we've uncovered these truths, we must decide if we want to share them or teach what we've realized in some way.

We all have a Master inside of us, whether we know it or not. Maybe you play the piano skillfully and want to teach others how to play. Perhaps you excel at the foxtrot and want to teach others to dance. Or perhaps you are a wiz at role-playing games like Dungeons & Dragons (for which you are literally called a Dungeon *Master*) and want to share that skill. You may guide people around the historical landmarks in your city. You may reveal the nuances of programming computers or lead others through the emotional labyrinth of coping with cancer. You may help others heal from heartbreak. There is almost no limit to the directions Master energy can take. All you need to do is own it and keep it in balance.

## The Master in Balance

One of the most important factors, if not *the* most important factor, in working and living from a place of balanced Master energy is maintaining healthy boundaries. In order to do this, you must know yourself well. You must be firm, but not rigid. You must be flexible, but not be a pushover. As you balance and access your Master energy, I can't stress enough how important it is to be in the moment, to stay present to your own self and to the people with whom you interact.

Those with balanced Master energy often become:

- Teachers

- Guides

- Leaders

- Mentors

- Truth-seekers

- Channelers of wisdom

Balanced Masters are typically:

- Open-minded

- Honest with themselves

- Introspective

- Nonideological

- Caring

- Calming

Balanced Masters gravitate toward activities in which they can shine a light so others can see.

To stay balanced, Masters must remain centered, fueled, protected, and aware of all the energies in the world that want to push, pull, use, squeeze, or manipulate them. We've all heard stories of gurus sleeping with their students or therapists losing objectivity with their clients. These stories all reflect a failure to maintain boundaries. But there are also subtler boundaries that Masters must establish and maintain, like not allowing crowds to get inside their heads energetically or not excessively opening their hearts to heal other people's pain at their own expense.

Boundaries are an expression of personal power, and healthy boundaries are an expression of healthy personal power. As a Master, don't be afraid to acknowledge your boundaries. They can be a lesson for others in and of themselves.

### The Master in Deficit

When I felt I had come out the other side on my spiritual journey after spending a year in India and seven years in Hawaii studying meditation and the healing arts, I began teaching more and more. Eventually, I decided to move to Upstate New York and start teaching for myself. Within a few years of putting my meditations online, they started gaining followers. I started getting daily messages of gratitude from all over the world. I also got deep, difficult questions from people about how to handle certain energies on their life path. This was difficult, of course, because I knew I couldn't answer their questions definitively most of the time. But I eventually realized that my job was to teach them tools so they could find their own answers.

Many of these questions related to a deficiency in Master energy. This deficit often manifests as:

- A lack of certainty

- Feelings of being an imposter

- Difficulty making decisions

- Seeking answers in others and ignoring the inner voice

- A constant need for a guru or guide

- Excessive reliance on the intellect

- Resistance to becoming a guide or mentor

- Denial that the truth is available to be understood

- A tendency to remain a student for too long

- Hiding from society

These traits generally stem from three main causes: feelings of unworthiness, an aversion to judgment, and excessive humility.

### The Imposter Syndrome

One of the great challenges for Masters is feeling that they are worthy. Many people who are awakening the Master energy in themselves are resistant to the idea of being someone else's teacher. They question their own knowledge and succumb to self-doubt. I call this the "imposter syndrome," a state of mind characterized by the belief that we are frauds merely pretending to be successful or enlightened or creative or knowledgeable. Sooner or later, we fear, someone is going to figure this out and expose us as charlatans.

These feelings of unworthiness affect us all. I don't think a day has gone by when I haven't fallen prey to imposter syndrome. And these thoughts are entirely natural. But at the same time, you need to remember that you are here to share your experiences, your wisdom. What you don't know, you simply don't know. And that's okay. As long as you're honest about that, you can let others decide whether you have value for them or not.

### Aversion to Judgment

Masters in deficit may also find themselves feeling an aversion to attention, because when people pay attention to them, they are seen and judged. They may not like the spotlight and the energy that comes from praise, but they must learn to manage that energy in a healthy way. They must accept that sharing their light with the world is part of their journey, and so are the ramifications of that attention.

As teachers or guides, we must learn what kind of praise to accept. And we also must learn what kind of criticism to accept. Some criticism can be incredibly constructive. On the other hand, some criticism can be laced with envy, anger, or unhealthy projection. Some people project, troll, hate, and want to make others feel small in order to make themselves feel better. As the yogi Sri Yuktiswar said: "Some people try to become tall by cutting off the heads of others." It's easy for those who lean toward a deficiency in Master energy to take judgment to heart and shrink away from their power.

### Excessive Humility

This aversion to judgment can also manifest as excessive humility. Those deficient in Master energy may put other teachers on pedestals and believe that they will never achieve that state themselves. When I was in college studying philosophy, I believed that I would never understand as much about life as my professors did, because they were so much smarter than I was. Because I believed that intellect equaled wisdom, I put my professors on pedestals. I did it again in India, where I revered all gurus, believing that I would never be as enlightened as they were.

Later, I realized that this attitude was rooted in excessive humility. But there is a fine line between humility and deficiency. Recognizing that you have the potential to become a Buddha in your own right doesn't necessarily come from the ego. It may come from understanding and experience. The ability to self-validate and find certainty in your own truth is essential to overcoming a deficiency in Master energy. All you have to do is examine the invalidation that is programmed into you by religion and society and resist the conviction that there is always someone who knows better.

## The Master in Excess

Excess Master energy can manifest in any psychological system where group members are essentially forced into doing things they don't want to. It can be seen in situations involving business leaders, corporations, political organizations, and sports—the CEO who is always right, the person who always needs to teach but never learns, the narcissistic guru with a God complex, the know-it-all professor, or the zealot who thinks everyone needs to believe what they believe. Unchecked, these energies can cause serious damage to both individuals and to society as a whole, as we have seen countless times throughout history.

It's often much easier to see overt forms of excess Master energy in others than it is to see them in ourselves. The signs may be subtle and difficult to recognize at first, which is why it's important to practice radical honesty and to work with these energies in depth. Some of these signs include:

- "The One" complex

- Overzealousness

- Being a know-it-all

- Speaking often, but not listening well

- Constantly trying to teach

- Being overly intellectual

- Arrogance

- A need for constant attention

- Manipulativeness

- Tendency to be power-hungry

- A need to be right

- Claiming to have a direct line to God

These imbalances are often grounded in two traits: emotional immaturity and self-aggrandizement.

### Emotional Immaturity

Many cults are born from an unhealthy and out-of-balance Master energy. These movements are often led by people who want to rise to their potential Master energy, but have become delusional, stuck, or misunderstood. These would-be leaders then abuse their positions and institute rigid rules and controls over their followers.

This sometimes happens when the person has had a deep spiritual experience and transformation, but has remained emotionally and psychologically immature. When life experience can't catch up to spiritual experience, Master energy can take over in an unhealthy way. I've seen countless spiritual teachers who may have had spiritual powers and insight, but were in desperate need of some humility, a good therapist, a grounding partner, or a kick in the ass.

### Self-Aggrandizement

I've personally witnessed gurus using legitimately powerful moments of precognitive awareness to elevate or promote themselves and lay claim to superior powers. But experiences like these don't make them Masters. They only affirm that all of life is connected in mysterious ways.

I've seen gurus engage in acts that I consider cruel, self-aggrandizing, and unnecessary. And I've seen gurus manipulate others and abuse their power. Gurus, it turns out, are people. And as in nearly every situation where people are involved, some are honest and compassionate, and some are manipulative and deceitful. None are perfect. That can make it challenging to know when a Master is genuine. But if you pay close attention to a person's energy, you can begin to tell the difference.

And of course, it's important to remember that even legitimate Masters will experience moments of deficiency and excess. We like to suppose that our leaders, gurus, mentors, and teachers are perfect. But the fact remains that they are people. And people are never perfect.

For example, I once had a guru that I *did* think was perfect. His energy was powerful and peaceful. You could feel it from the other side of the room. And I had many incredible healing experiences during the time I spent with him. He lived in a small room in an ashram in the Himalayas that was plagued by monkeys who were often aggressive and stole food. When he emerged from his room, however, they seemed to bow and back away.

One day, this guru was giving a deep and profound talk when someone asked a question that he didn't like. All of the sudden, he became visibly upset and snapped at us, saying: "If you don't like my teachings, then I'll go back to my room and won't come out anymore. I don't need to be here!" This experience was upsetting to me because, at the time, I still believed that perfection was possible and that there were teachers who were perfect.

Although many of my experiences were with Indian gurus, I want to be clear that every religious tradition in the world has leaders who are susceptible to an excess or perversion of Master energy. All leaders in all spheres are human.

## Back to Balance

Masters in balance understand that great healing, insight, and awakening arise from inner work and that it is the universe moving through them that is the source of their power, not themselves. Humility in the face of this truth is often a sign of an authentic teacher. When Master energy awakens and begins to reach its potential, it recognizes that whatever it's sharing or teaching, love is the underlying principle and the guiding force.

Whether balanced Masters are reaching out to ten people or ten million, they do so with care and purpose. As you develop into your Master energy, you will realize that it's less about the information, ideas, or strategies you are conveying than it is about the exchange of energy. That's why two people can say exactly the same thing, yet one transforms lives and the other is left with an empty tip jar. It's the energy behind the Master that matters.

Masters learn by teaching. Just as Creators are balanced by creating and Lovers heal by loving, Masters unfold their energy by sharing and guiding. Every class that I've ever taught has challenged me to go deeper into the topic I was teaching and to reconcile more of that energy in myself.

### Meditation to Balance Master Energy

This meditation can help you to balance your inner Master and harness its energy.

**Step 1:** Begin by recognizing where in your life you are ready to harness Master energy, and how you would like to apply it. Are you ready to lead? To teach? To mentor in some way? Are you ready to tackle self-knowledge and certainty?

**Step 2:** If you feel unsure, perhaps you are ready to take a step toward clarity of vision. If you are feeling enthusiastic about sharing your light, maybe you are ready to guide the way for others. Begin with what you see, sense, and feel without any judgment. There is nothing negative here—only signs pointing to your next step.

**Step 3:** What is that next step for you? See if you can be courageous enough to look at it with honest eyes and own it for yourself.

**Step 4:** What do you look like when you harness this energy? How does your life unfold? Can you feel that energy in this moment?

**Step 5:** Allow yourself to feel a sense of certainty and knowingness here. You don't need to know how everything is going to turn out, just that you feel and know your next step deeply. There is something in you that you would like to harness and share with the world.

**Step 6:** Finally, bring your awareness to the top of your head. From this energetically sensitive place, imagine that a color arises on top of your head that truly represents your Master energy in this moment. What is that color? How does it feel?

**Step 7:** Embrace yourself as a Master. You are in this life to develop your Master energy and help others in some way. Without fear or invalidation, recognize your true nature. With a deep connection to the other six energies, you are a true Master of yourself. Own it. Live it. Become it.

### Master Self-Reflection

Follow this meditation with some deep self-reflection. To help identify your deficient Master tendencies, ask yourself these questions:

- Do you have a hard time being certain and making decisions?

- Do you succumb to "imposter syndrome" when it comes to what you want to share with the world?

- Do you have a hard time hearing your inner voice or listening to your intuition?

- Do you often look to others for your answers?

- Do you avoid being a leader or guide for others when you know it's your time?

Now ask yourself these questions to help identify you excessive Master tendencies:

- When you come to a deep realization, do you need to convince everyone around you of it?

- Do you tend to speak too much and not listen enough?

- Do you sometimes experience a kind of certainty that comes from your ego?

- Do you sometimes inflate your own self-importance and want others to notice you?

- Do you often feel the need to be right or convince others that you are right?

Finally, consider these questions as you work to cultivate balanced Master energy:

- What holds me back from embracing my own inner Master? What are one or two things I can do to release those holds?

- Was there a moment in my life when someone invalidated me and made me lose certainty in myself? What would I say to that person?

- If I were a guide or mentor for others, in what way would I like to help them? Which of my other energies would I employ?

- What Masters in history do I admire and what are some of the qualities in them that I appreciate? If I could invite two of them to dinner, what would I ask them? What would I tell them about myself and my journey?

### Master Goals

Consider the difference between how Master energy works internally and externally. Then see if you can come up with three ways in which you can apply your Master energy to your life on an internal level. For example:

- Develop more certainty.

- Recognize my true self.

- Deepen into my intuition.

Now write down three ways in which you can apply your Master energy to your life on an external level. For example:

- Live by example.

- Be a mentor or guide to those I can help.

• Share my knowledge and wisdom through teaching and writing.

### Master Action: Teaching Others

As I mentioned at the beginning of the chapter, you don't have to be a spiritual leader to cultivate your Master energy. All you need to do is own your talents and truths and be prepared to share them with the world.

It can help to start small. If you have been telling yourself that you can't possibly have anything of worth to offer to the world, or if you have ideas that you'd like to share but have been too afraid to put out there, leave that aside for a moment. Instead, take out your journal and spend some time making a list of things you know how to do—skills in which you feel utterly confident. Keep these relatively small and simple—though if grander ideas occur to you, write them down too. Do you know how to bake a loaf of bread? Have you spent several years reading up on Greek mythology? Have you ever successfully planted tomatoes? Do you know how baseball statistics work? You may be surprised at how many things you come up with. But even if it's just one or two, that's sufficient.

Choose one of these skills and commit to teaching it to someone who would like to learn. Break it down into pieces and consider how you would teach it to someone who is a complete beginner. Ask a few friends and see if perhaps they'd like to spend an hour learning something new. Or if you're feeling adventurous and have the skill set, consider making a few video tutorials and posting them online. When your lesson is over, ask your students for feedback on your teaching abilities. How can you make the subject clearer? More exciting? More user-friendly? More practical? Then teach it again and see if you feel differently than you did the first time.

You are a guiding force of light in this world, and you are ready to share your wisdom and experience to help others along the path. That path may lead to spiritual enlightenment, but it may just as powerfully lead to homegrown tomatoes and a fresh-baked loaf of bread.

# Chapter 10

# The Soul in Balance

*Through our eyes, the universe is perceiving itself.*
*Through our ears, the universe is listening to its harmonies.*
*We are the witnesses through which the universe*
*becomes conscious of its glory, of its magnificence.*

—Alan Watts

In 326 BC, Alexander the Great invaded India in his quest to conquer the world. It's said that he once came across a naked yogi and stopped to talk. Indian mythologist Devdutt Pattanaik imagined what their conversation might have been like in his popular TED Talk "East vs. West."

Alexander finds the naked yogi sitting still on a rock and asks him: "Why are you just sitting there? What are you doing with your life?"

"I'm focusing on nothingness," the yogi responds.

Alexander laughs and says: "What a waste of a life."

"What are you doing with your life?" the yogi asks.

"Conquering the world!" Alexander replies.

To which the yogi responds: "What a waste of a life."

Pattanaik imagined that the two men laughed, each thinking the other crazy. I see in this moment an important and symbolic meeting of the Eastern and Western minds—two sides of the same coin that we all have inside of us. And the difference in their perspectives is crucial. It lies in their conceptions of time.

For Alexander, time is linear; it has a beginning and an end. You must conquer life before it is too late; you must become a hero like Achilles and other figures from Greek mythology. For the yogi, life is cyclical. You are reborn again and again, until you learn certain lessons. There is no reason to conquer anything. It's a futile exercise in vanity. When you reach one mountaintop, you will look out across the horizon and find that there are an infinite number of them.

In Indian philosophy, the world we live in, the world of form, is known by its Sanskrit name, *maya*—which means "illusion." We go through what the Hindus call *samsara*—cycles of endless births and deaths that go on and on until we break the chain. As I went deeper into this philosophy in my early twenties, I started to disdain the material world and the people who thought it was important.

But I have also experienced the world from Alexander's perspective. There have been times in my life when I found myself being ambitious, focused on progress and on building my business, and wanting to conquer the world in my own way. Then I realized that I had personal needs and desires that I had shoved deep down into my unconscious. I started thinking about having a relationship, building a family, owning a home, and possessing the financial means to be independent.

At times, I felt as if I were at war with myself—the spiritual and material parts of me battling for supremacy, pulling me in different directions. My spiritual side told me that self-realization was all that mattered; my human side said: "I'm hungry!"

We all have both Alexander and the yogi inside us. And the tension we feel between these two worlds is no accident. In fact, that friction is useful. If approached correctly, it can light a healthy fire in us.

Balancing the seven energies of the soul is about finding peace and equilibrium between the Alexander and the yogi in you—between mastering the external world of matter and understanding the internal world of energy. As you step into each of the seven energies of the soul, you start to recognize where there is conflict in yourself that needs healing and give yourself permission to embrace the entire spectrum of life.

As the Creator, the Healer, the Artist, or any other energy archetype begins to reach its potential in you, you may find a tension between the practical worldly energies and the idealistic, ethereal, or spiritual ones. These two forces can actually complement each other instead of being in competition. In fact, they *must* work together if you're going to find happiness and balance in life.

## Integration and Harmony

Now that we've walked through each energy and meditated together, I want to emphasize again that no energy type is an island unto itself. To be successful and fulfilled in life—to be fully functioning in mind, body, and soul—all your energies must be integrated and work together in balance, complementing each other.

I once had the opportunity to work with the successful CEO of an innovative tech start-up. We were discussing her vision and leadership style. She had built an amazing company, but she still felt that something was missing in the organization.

As we dove into her own personal journey, she realized that, through her upbringing and her Ivy League education, she had been taught to lead from a very intellectual and calculated place. Her Creator, Explorer, and Master energies were very strong. The missing piece was her Lover energy. She realized that, if she could weave the fabric of compassion and love through her company and make sure her team could sense that they were on a mission together, the entire organization would be better off. She committed to opening her heart more and sharing that love with her employees. It was beautiful to watch the shift.

I also had a friend who was a very talented therapist. One day, he decided he wanted to leave the organization in which he worked and go to work for himself. Then he decided to write a book. He utilized his Healer energies as a therapist, his Master energies as a guide, his Creator energies as a business owner, and his Artist energies as a writer. This led him to find balance and integration in his life.

A great example of what it looks like when someone balances all seven energies is Oprah Winfrey. She is undeniably a strong Creator and Explorer with multiple businesses and commercial interests. She is a Master who guides others in many different emotional and spiritual areas. Her Healer and Lover energies are evident in her charitable work. Her sense of personal style and presence demonstrate her Artist energy. And her discipline and determination display strong Warrior energy. Thus she is a great example of integration and balance in all seven areas. Is she perfect? Of course not; she's human. But she clearly isn't afraid of living up to her potential in every area of life.

### Meditation to Balance the Seven Energies

Now that you've explored each of the seven energies in turn, where do you see yourself lacking integration and balance? How can you find harmony? This meditation may help you to integrate your energies and achieve that balance.

**Step 1:** Stepping into your interior world as you close your physical eyes, notice your mind's eye begin to open. In front of you, imagine that there are seven roses, each a different color, all lined up in a row. Each rose represents one energy of the soul. Moving from left to right, you have the Creator, the Healer, the Warrior, the Lover, the Artist, the Explorer, and the Master.

**Step 2:** As you look at all seven roses, take a moment to scan them to see which ones seem full of energy and color and which ones look depleted and needing more of your attention and energy.

**Step 3:** Take note of which energy or energies seem the least integrated into who you are. Perhaps you even feel a bit alienated from these parts of your soul.

**Step 4:** Take the rose that seems as if it needs attention in this moment, and touch it to your heart center in the middle of your chest. You'll know which rose it is because it will wiggle a bit or move in some way. Or you may just experience a knowingness.

**Step 5:** As you touch this rose to your heart, you may get an image or a feeling around why you've been avoiding this energy or what kind of care, healing, and attention it needs.

**Step 6:** See if you can give it that attention. Then do this for any other roses that seem to need care. Take as long as you need to do this.

**Step 7:** When you're feeling complete, notice all seven roses, all seven energies of the soul, vibrating in harmony. Then watch as they merge into one rose. Take that rose and bring it into your heart. Let it dissolve into your being. Integrate all seven energies and feel their balance in your being.

Take some time to jot down how your body and mind feel after this meditation. Refreshed? Energized? I hope so. If not, try journaling a bit about which of the roses is a tight bud or perhaps beyond its prime. You may want to do a meditation on that energy.

Then treat yourself. Go out and buy yourself seven beautiful roses. Find as many varied colors as you can. Or get big juicy red ones or beautiful calming white ones or cheerful and healing yellow ones—whatever color appeals to you. Put them in a vase in your meditation space and admire them.

You've done incredible work on this journey. Know that the journey isn't over, however. Whenever you find yourself stuck, lost, uncertain, or looking for answers, tap into each energy and ask it to show you your next steps in life.

# Conclusion

## Next Steps

At the beginning of our journey together, I told you that the seven energies of the soul came from the seven most commonly asked common questions I've heard from my students over the years. In reality, however, every question my students asked was essentially the same one in different forms: *What is my next step?* To find that next step, you have to know yourself and understand what you value.

Whether you are stuck on a relationship, having a career problem, wrestling with a creative block, or experiencing an existential meltdown, it always comes down to the same thing: What do you do next? How do you know what the right next step really is? Is there even such a thing as a right next step?

When we struggle with these questions, we often turn to others for answers—a partner, a parent, an expert, a spiritual teacher or healer, or even the Internet. But the truth is that no one can answer our deepest questions in life for us—the ones that hit closest to home. Is this person the right partner for me? Is it my path to move to that city? What is my purpose in life? The Buddha had to leave all of his teachers, sit, and find his answers for himself. So do you.

We all have to find the courage to look within. Otherwise, no matter what the answers are, they may not really sink in and integrate with our soul. We may wake up after this dream of a life ends, look down at our decisions, and recognize that they were right on paper, but lacked the real depth that we were searching for.

Like T. S. Eliot, I want to end our journey where we began—with the idea that our answers are born out of our energy. When our energy shifts, when we truly flower, our answers also flower. They aren't static mental images. Our answers are alive. They're expressions of growth that emanate from a soul that is reaching its potential.

To awaken your soul in this life, you have to be willing to look at those painful places where you are stuck and heal them. But you must also learn how to look. Through our meditations together, you've explored each energy. Now you must balance and integrate those energies into a fulfilling and purposeful life.

Our deepest answers come to us from a realm beyond intellect, and even beyond feeling. They land in our mind's eye and in our heart when we open to life and to healing. As you quiet your mind, get in touch with your heart, ground your values, and own each soul energy, your answers will begin to emerge. What you do with those answers and how you choose to share yourself with the world are up to you. The best advice I can give you is to quit hiding, quit underperforming, quit running from your potential, and get out there and be who you were born to be. The rest of the world needs you.

Many spiritual traditions teach that, when we die, we experience what's called a life review. And there are only two metrics that really matter in this review: how much you loved and how much you learned. Any worthwhile experience that is aligned to your deeper purpose will bring you both love and wisdom. And those two things—love and wisdom—will pour out of your being and touch the people around you. Misery loves company, but so does love and growth.

So own the seven energies of your soul—and get to work!

## Acknowledgments

There was a time in my life when I thought I had to do everything on my own to prove myself to the world—that was called my twenties. I was arrogant about my own enlightenment and what that path was supposed to look like. The irony of that is not lost on me. There was a point when I realized there was a difference between waking up and growing up, and this book is hopefully a reflection of that insight. And to grow up spiritually, I needed a lot of help—perhaps more than most.

When I first sat down to write these acknowledgments, I remembered the saying, "The bigger the dream, the bigger the team." And that has definitely been true in my life experience. We often think of our personal growth as a solitary process, but for me, without the influence of all of my teachers, healers, coaches, guides, colleagues, and friends, I would probably be playing small, hiding from the world, and holding my insights close to my chest. I needed people to see me and validate my potential before I was ready to do it myself.

So I want to acknowledge, with the deepest of gratitudes, all the people who helped me loosen my grip on those insights and share them with the world.

But before I get to those folks, I want to start by acknowledging my students. It's their struggles, their feedback, their inspiration, and their love that have truly fueled me to continue teaching and sharing. There is nothing more fulfilling to me in this life than seeing someone take a tool that I taught, find their own answers and insights with it, and transform pain into wisdom.

So to anyone who has ever sat with me to meditate, laughed at a bad joke of mine in class, or read through this book and applied it to your life, from the deepest place in my soul, thank you for doing the work and being open. I'm not interested in being your guru, but your friend, and occasionally your guide.

I also want to thank my publisher Randy Davila, for helping shape this book, sharpen its clarity, and for all the hard work it took to publish it. And for inviting me into the Insight Events USA family to teach retreats and events.

To Sara Sutterfield Winn, Melissa Kirk, and Jan Johnson for their amazing work as editors and for being patient with me . . .

To my friend and author, Scott Stabile, who synchronistically popped into my life at the exact moment I was ready to write a book with his advice and insights . . .

To Jona, who has managed everything I do from the back end, and who keeps my wild creative self on track . . .

To the team at the Insight Timer meditation app, for sharing my work with the world and for doing business with so much integrity . . .

To my family and friends for being so supportive as I took the most crooked of life paths, traveling, searching, teaching, and building. And particularly to all four of my grandparents, who against all odds survived the Holocaust and brought our family to the United States in 1979 to find opportunity . . .

To all my co-teachers and friends that give me inspiration, including Cody Edner and Marjorie Bratt-Gomero . . .

And to all future souls that may read this who need a bit of direction and structure on their life path . . . From the bottom of my Lover's heart, my Creator's hands, my Warrior's spirit, and my Healer's gratitude, thank you.

# About the Author

David Gandelman is a spiritual teacher, author, and guide, whose mission is to awaken souls on their path of growing into being human, and living an enlightened, purpose-driven life.

He is the founder of the Meditation School app, and host of the Meditation School, Energy Matters, and Grounded Sleep podcasts. And his meditations have been streamed millions of times. He has taught at Cornell University, NBC Universal, SAP, and numerous other organizations.

David holds a B.A. in Western philosophy from Rutgers University, which combined with his studies in Eastern spiritual traditions living in the Himalayas, as well as his experience as the director of a school for intuitive development and mysticism in Hawaii, informs a teaching style that connects energetic experience, ancient wisdom traditions, and humor in order to create a safe atmosphere for people interested in learning to meditate and develop into their potential.

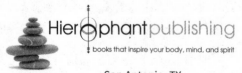

Hier◯phant publishing
books that inspire your body, mind, and spirit

San Antonio, TX
www.hierophantpublishing.com